CONTENTS

CHAPTER 3:

INTRODUCTION

D o you ever sit back and ask why it appears almost impossible for you to achieve your fitness goals even after exercising regularly and following all the instructions on a diet? Well, if it makes you feel any better, you are not alone. Yes, there are thousands of people who have asked the same question at different times, which means they are or were in your shoes at some point. However, the good news is that the answer to this question isn't far-fetched.

As human beings, we are often too engrossed with different aspects of our lives, such as family, career, education, etc. As a result, we forget to look out for our health until we notice some evident problems. When we begin to notice these problems, there is a clear difference between our current state of health, how healthy we used to be, or how healthy we should be. We then attempt to find the fastest and most effective way to correct, albeit with superficial research that appears to have the proposed "solutions." However, it becomes an issue for many to worry about only when they don't experience the results they anticipate as and when due.

It is almost natural that we become too focused on the end goals that we ignore the process and certain essential health factors like body type. Surprisingly, this is one factor that has an impact on other factors. You may not have heard or read about body types, and if you already have, you might be forced to ask how it relates to the problem at hand. It might interest you to know that your body type is a fundamental factor determining your weight loss, weight gain, and overall health journey. Now that you already have an idea of this, you are probably itching to know more.

Commonly, people in their mid-twenties and older often struggle with poor health following their chain of daily activities that leave them with barely any time to go through any form of the fitness journey, especially the common ones - exercise and a healthy diet. However, there hasn't been much of a difference for some others who have adopted methods to combat poor health. If you fall under any of these categories, your frustrations are understandable, which is why this book is highly recommended for you.

The sole purpose of this book is to provide clarity and educate young and busy adults on essential factors that are usually the bedrock for healthy living. Unfortunately, most people are ignorant of these factors and their critical role in living a healthy life.

Therefore, we will start this book by discussing body types. You will get to know the different classifications of body types, how each works, and the science behind them. These will be presented with pictorial illustrations to aid understanding and ensure clarity. Also, this book will provide you with a brief background of how these body types came into being. It will also discuss the pathological differences between these body types at length. You will learn how to deal with combined or mixed body types. This book will also help individuals who are aware of their body type but need help altering their current state.

Having understood body types, another important aspect that should be of concern is what you eat. Ordinarily, people refer to dieting as rationalizing food portions to control their physical appearance or avoid health issues. This definition isn't entirely wrong, but at the same time, it isn't quite true. A healthy diet is an integral part of healthy living, and it varies from one person to another. This is why many people feel that the eating pattern they have adopted isn't providing them with the results they want or expect.

Often, the problem isn't from the diet; the eating pattern in question isn't suitable for them. Therefore, this book will introduce you to different healthy diets that are suitable for your unique body type. It will also provide a meal plan for each of the discussed body types, making it easier for you to enjoy your meals without fear of adverse effects.

Just like adopting a healthy diet, exercise is an essential aspect of keeping fit. Exercise does not always have to be strenuous. However, it is important to choose workout patterns that are suitable for your unique body type. Therefore, after reading this book, you will have gathered more knowledge about the various physical activities and choose suitable options for yourself.

Another important aspect of the discussion in this book is genetics and its effect on the human body. Common genetic factors such as age, family, health issues, etc., will be discussed at length to broaden your knowledge of handling these factors.

Intermittent fasting is a trending topic in the health world today. It is highly recommendable for people who are too busy to indulge in workouts or patient enough to rationalize meals in different proportions. This book will provide more information on how to remain healthy through intermittent fasting by discussing what it is, how it works, and how it can be implemented for your body type with the proper understanding.

In conclusion, this book will educate and clarify the aspects that you are not doing correctly for those that have adopted various methods to ensure healthy living and for those that are yet to start; it will highlight the steps to take to begin this worthwhile journey.

CHAPTER 1:
INTRODUCTION TO SOMATOLOGY

As a branch of the humanities, somatology is defined as examining or studying the human body. It is derived from the Latin word somatologia, which means "to study the human body." Physicalism also describes it as the study of material bodies or substances. According to ancient writers, the human body is made up of three parts: body, brain, and soul — soma, mind, and pneuma.

Somatology is, in one sense, the physical and physiological study of the entire body, intending to determine how the various body parts interact. However, it can also refer to the properties of living organic entities. Somatologists study a wide range of topics related to the human body and how it functions.

Historical Development Of Somatotype

Renowned American psychologist William Herbert Sheldon coined the word somatotypes to describe different body types. He was a specialist and therapist in the mid-20th century, with degrees from Brown University and the

University of Colorado. He also attended Harvard and Columbia Universities. He first proposed his ideas for a three-component rating scheme for assessing human shape in the book - Varieties of Human Physique.

According to him, somatotype is made up of:

> **Endomorph** - characterized by a relative predominance of soft roundness throughout the body.
> **Ectomorph** - characterized by a predominance of linearity and fragility.
> **Mesomorph** - characterized by a relative predominance of muscle, bone, and connective tissue.

The somatotype was an assessment of a person's body shape regardless of their size. It was assumed from the study that irrespective of changes in appearance, a person's somatotype remained the same throughout their lives. Thus, W.H. Sheldon's method is by far the most adaptable, accurate, and thorough.

Tanner summarized Sheldon's system as arduous and time-consuming and mentioned that the investigators ran into unexpected challenges trying to adopt this metric technique for several years and have had many problems.

In 1954, Sheldon, alongside other scholars, distributed his Atlas of Men. This Atlas included photos of over a thousand men. In addition, it contained refreshed stature weight tables for men from 18 to 63 years of age.

Another interesting evaluation that Sheldon pointed out in the Atlas was the impact of sex, age, and nutrition on somatotype. Also, a notable gesture of Sheldon was his attempt to make it possible for other interested researchers to use his organized rating system to assess human shape. His efforts aimed to provide an explanation rather than a change in his fundamental position regarding the concept of somatotype.

In his definition, Sheldon pointed out the following basic characteristics of a somatotype:

➢ The somatotype is a shape rating rather than size assessment.

➢ It is made up of Endomorph, Ectomorph, and Mesomorph.

➢ The total number of pieces in the three portions is supposed to be between 9 and 12.

➢ Each of the three sections is used in equal and irregular amounts to create a subject's body.

➢ A subject's somatotype does not vary over time or with health conditions when appropriately assessed.

In 1954, Parnell published a work that outlined a method for determining the relative strength of somatotype parts within a subject. However, Parnell's diagrams of somatotype in his 1958 book were entirely based on anthropometry.

A few experts examined the relationship between anthropometric amounts and somatotype parts, while others compared photogrammetry (estimations from photos) to anthropometry (direct estimates of the subject).

Heath and Carter published a definitive analysis of Heath's 1963 technique and Parnell's 1958 somatotype determination strategy in 1966. These four explicit changes are articulations of the following fundamental premises:

➢ The somatotype strategy should be as reliable as possible.

➢ For all ages and genders, internal consistency dictates that the same rating strategy and scale be used.

➢ The somatotype is a representation of the current shape rather than a morphogenotype indicator.

➢ Somatotyping's unique "jargon" should be protected to the greatest extent possible.

In 1967, Petersen issued an Atlas for Somatotyping Children, but it did not offer a considerable discussion of the approach for evaluating the somatotype of children or the specific challenges associated with somatotyping children, as Sheldon's map book did.

Preston and Singh developed a sophisticated device for photographing somatotype using light moving through a cutoff, size-changed subject slide. The creators claim that this method of determining somatotype is far easier than other methods currently in use.

Tallness and skinfolds were factored into the computations for the three somatotypes, depending on the subject's somatotype. Thus, the conclusion was that although larger people have larger skinfolds than smaller people of similar shapes, both should receive the same endomorph rating for body shape. Heath and Carter have supported this.

Carter was the first to distribute conditions via Carter in 1980, allowing direct prediction of Heath-Carter somatotype from anthropometric parameters without the use of tables.

However, the Heath-Carter somatotype (either the table method or the conditions) is used in logical reports to use somatotyping. Furthermore, the Heath-Carter somatotype is the accepted norm for current somatotype assurance, according to the 1982 Perceived Somatotype Scale.

Classification of Somatotype

There are different ways to classify the physiological body in the same way that character types group certain examples of behavior into personalities. Understanding the various physiological body types will help you better understand how yours works. Individuals enjoy and find comfort in being able to relate to others when they understand their own characteristics and mental processes better. The human body is as much a product of bias and behavior as it is of DNA and hereditary traits, which leads us to the three different classifications of body types. They are Hormonal body types, Ayurvedic types, and Structural types.

Knowing what your body type is will help you better understand the following:

- Healthy diet recommendations and meal plans for you.
- Exercise recommendations for your body type.
- Why your body structure appears the way it does.
- Weight/fat loss plans.
- Weight gain plans.
- Common health risks associated with body type.
- How to deal with potential health risks.

Hormonal Body Types

According to the hormonal theory, four basic body types are defined by how an individual transports fat. This could either be by storing it in equal amounts in their stomach or the lower part of their body. What's intriguing about the hormonal type hypothesis is that it explains why many people might lose weight and exercise in the same way but have different results.

Recent research has proven that changes in the elements of our organs may affect body form, which is often a result of the accumulation of excess fat or liquid. Therefore, working on the necessary organs of your body can help model the body to its appropriate shape.

The Four basic body types under this heading are:

- **Adrenal:** This is the chemical cortisol responsible for weight gain in the stomach and back. People with this body type usually have a round appearance. They believe that regardless of how much they exercise or reduce their carb intake, it is nearly impossible to lose weight around their waist. This is because the weight is caused by a substance that effectively uses proteins and fats in the lower legs before storing them in the mid-section of the body. Exercising might make it more difficult for people with Adrenal bodies to lose weight since they are now under pressure, which is what is driving them to store fat in the first place. However, it is important to note that people with Adrenal bodies won't be able to change unless they deal with whatever underlying mental tensions they are experiencing.

➢ **Thyroid:** This is responsible for making it either indisputably tough to get more fit or challenging to maintain weight. People under this category will generally store weight evenly but fluctuate, sometimes gaining a lot of weight in a short period for no apparent cause.

➢ **Liver:** This body type is caused by the body's inability to cope with excessive ingestion of alcoholic beverages or processed foods. The Liver body type is most commonly depicted as someone with a "paunch," or someone who stores all of their weight in front of their waist. As a result, the weight will be imbalanced compared to the rest of their body, and they will have a tendency to put on

INTRODUCTION TO SOMATOLOGY

excess weight relative to their body frame. People
with this body type should note that diet
adjustments, particularly the elimination or
reduction of alcohol consumption, can often help
with weight loss.

> **Ovary:** This body type is symbolized by the volatile
  nature of estrogen production. This feature doesn't
  apply to men. It is similar to people who store
  weight in their lower stomach, lower back, hips,
  and thighs. Individuals in this category are more
  likely to experience adverse effects during their
  period, and they may struggle with water retention
  and weariness. In addition, contraception
  medication has a significant impact on their daily
  well-being.

Ayurvedic Body Type

Also known as Doshas. It is based on the idea that bodies
are made up of a mix of elements like everything else in
nature. The Doshas reflect the various ways in which bodies
evolve using the four basic elements of water, air, fire, and
earth. These elements may not be accurately measured, but
they can be easily observed.

The Ayurvedic body types are:

> **Pitta:** The two main components of this are fire and
  water. The typical features of its appearance are:
  evenly proportioned, medium edge, a few parts
  stronger than others, may effectively overheat or

hold water. Common attributes of Pittas are Determination and Coordination. People under this category like to be busy and achieve goals and are infamous for causing problems when there is nothing to gain.

➢ **Vata:** The two primary components of this category are air and water. The typical features of its appearance are: tall with long appendages and cold on a daily basis. In addition, people under this category are usually sensitive, quickly taken off track, touchy, despise schedules and spend time daydreaming.

➢ **Kapha:** The main components are earth and water. The typical features of its appearance are: occasional overweight, large form, effectively holds fat while being quite fantastic and athletic. People under this category are usually enthusiastic about life, exceptional at connecting, prefer a more sedentary way of life, enjoy relaxing and appreciating life.

Structural Body Types

W.H Sheldon propounded this classification of body types in his research in the 1940s. People fall into three main body types, each explaining how they will react to diet and activities in general. These three basic body types explain appetite, metabolic capability, and natural tendency to retain weight and fat.

The three body types under this classification are:

> **Ectomorph:** People in this category are usually small and delicate. They can eat whatever they want without gaining weight. They don't expend many calories and can struggle to build muscle when needed. They are usually quite tall, but they don't have to be. Examples of people with ectomorph body types are Models and athletes.

> **Endomorph:** Endomorphs are the polar opposite of ectomorphs in that they are often more prone to store fat. They have a hard time losing weight and have low muscle tone. They have strong food desires and usually struggle to regulate their eating. They are prone to being overweight and are typically heavier than others due to their heavier bone structure.

> **Mesomorph:** They have a generally balanced physique, a small abdomen, a low muscle-to-fat ratio, and are easily put on muscle. They find it easy to lose weight when they need to, and they often have smaller appetites. Mesomorphs can occasionally be classified as both ectomorphs and endomorphs because, in many instances, they may have features of both. In any case, they are distinct from both of those groups because losing or gaining weight is not a very difficult task for them.

Although it is not surprising that most people fall into one of these categories, it is not difficult to fit into a variety of them. However, for the purpose of this book, we will focus on the structural body types.

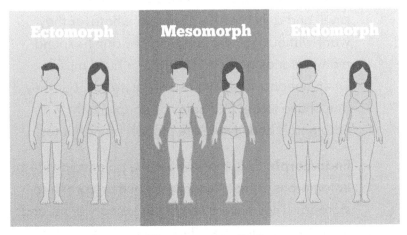

Ectomorph   Mesomorph   Endomorph

Photo source: mPort

The above is a pictorial illustration of the male and female structural body types as classified by Sheldon.

As human beings, our skeletal frame and body configuration determine our acquired body type. However, the notion is that everyone falls into one of these three structural body types and that, in some cases, some people possess traits from two or even all three somatotypes. Therefore, individuals can also be divided into somatotypes based on their morphologies: square, hourglass, triangle, or round.

Nutritionists, practicing physiologists, specialists, and even fitness experts have used the concept of somatotypes introduced by Sheldon to help them create an appealing and effective fitness plan. Hence, we will extensively discuss the three types under this classification below.

Ectomorph

Ectomorphs are recognized to be humans with slim and fit bodies. They have a modest bone structure with shoulders that are smaller than their hips in general. Although people with the ectomorph body type are usually regarded as "extremely fortunate," being an ectomorph does come with its own set of challenges.

One of these challenges is the misleading appearance. For example, even though ectomorphs appear to be slim, they may have a low muscle-to-fat ratio. So, in some cases, they may appear underweight on the surface. Also, as ectomorphs get older, their ability to digest food quickly slows down, resulting in weight gain that they aren't used to.

Whatever the case may be, being an ectomorph does not imply prolonged weakness. You can be as strong and healthy as someone with a different body type, but the focus should be on a large eating plan and modified activity.

Some of the notable characteristics of Ectomorphs are:

➢ They struggle to gain weight regardless of how much carbs or fats they consume.
➢ They have long arms and smaller muscles, which defines their appearance
➢ They are skinny and lean
➢ They have a small bone structure
➢ Their shoulders are narrower than their hips

> ➤ They have a small chest and buttocks
> ➤ They can eat anything they want without gaining excess weight.
> ➤ They experience fast metabolism.
> ➤ They easily lose muscle mass.
> ➤ They have a medium height, especially women

Endomorph

If a person believes that it is challenging for them to lose weight, they most likely have an endomorphic body type. Endomorphs have a high muscle-to-fat ratio and quickly gain fat and struggle to lose weight. The endomorphic body structure is commonly referred to as "three-sided."

Endomorphs often have more muscle than ectomorphs and mesomorphs; however, this is usually accompanied by a high muscle-to-fat ratio. They also have a slower metabolism, which is why endomorphs gain weight quickly and need to work hard in the gym to lose fat rather than muscle.

Some of the notable characteristics of Endomorphs are:

> ➤ Lack of muscle definition
> ➤ They usually experience a slow metabolic rate
> ➤ They carry a lot of weight in their thighs, buttocks, and hips
> ➤ They have a large bone structure
> ➤ Unlike the other body types, they have shorter arms and legs, as well as small hands and feet

> ➤ They struggle to lose weight

Mesomorph

For diverse reasons, this body type is believed to be the optimum body type. Usually, mesomorphs possess traits from both Ectomorphy and Endomorphy.

A mesomorph is a person who has an athletic build. Although they may easily gain both fat and muscle, they will burn fat more quickly than ectomorphs and endomorphs while maintaining muscle mass.

The body is typically wider at the shoulders, narrow at the hips, and noticeably lower waistline than the other body types.

Some of the notable characteristics of Mesomorphs are:

> ➤ They have an efficient metabolism
> ➤ For mesomorphs, gaining muscle and losing fat are both relatively simple tasks.
> ➤ They react quickly to exercise
> ➤ They have shoulders that are wider than their hips
> ➤ They are naturally slim
> ➤ They have an athletic build
> ➤ They have a medium bone structure
> ➤ They have defined muscle

CHAPTER 2:
GENETICS, METABOLISM, AND HORMONES

Looking closely at the kind of life we live where we eat processed food, sit for prolonged periods, drive from one location to the other without walking, it shouldn't come as a shock that weight-related health issues are on the rise. Although some people spend so much on diet plans, there is hardly any difference.

Sometimes, our bodies are responsible for a portion of our health-related problems, if not most of them. For instance, let's take into consideration a machine. Each component of a machine impacts the other components to work efficiently. We can compare the human body to a machine that requires a great deal of attention. The body is continually assessing and changing itself in response to information from both within and outside. And just like a machine, all the parts of the body work together. Hence, if one part of the machine (body) fails, it is possible that other parts may fail as well.

This chapter will discuss some of the basic factors that influence our physique. Primarily, we would discuss the aspects linked with genetics (hormones and metabolic changes) to educate about factors that influence body weight, hunger, body composition, and metabolism.

Genetics

While on vacation with her friends, Bella walked up to Samantha and expressed her concerns about her future. One of her concerns was her uncertainty about her physical appearance in ten years. Samantha smiled and replied with "just take a look at your mom, and you will find the answer to your question." Many people who will agree with Samantha will do so based on their understanding of genetics and how it impacts our physique. However, for those who do not understand, this section will explain it.

According to various studies, genetics determines everything in a person, starting from the most minute details such as hair color to significant ones such as chronic diseases. A person's genes play a role in determining important details such as where they store body fat. Hence, this may have serious health implications on the person, especially in cases where there is an indicator that there is a lot of stored fat. This can increase the risk of cardiovascular diseases and diabetes. Following additional medical research, new medication targeting such genetic polymorphisms to help prevent obesity may become available.

Hormones and Genes

Generally, when we think about genetics, we think of the characteristics we inherit from our parents. However, as we grow older, we may begin to notice additional characteristics that we may have inherited from our parents, such as hair color, eye color, face shape, etc. In addition, our hormones, particularly our thyroid hormones, are influenced by the way DNA operates.

Everything in your body is dictated by the genes you were born with. This ranges from your growth to your internal processes and even your body's ability to make hormones. Hormones have the ability to alter every organ and system in the human body. However, genes play an essential role in the production of hormones.

Hormones have been found to have the potential to activate genes. As a result, our genetic composition determines the way we are constructed and how we function. These hormones can become unpredictable as we grow older. If your body's hormones are imbalanced, your cells will be unable to work properly. In women, for example, low estrogen levels can change how your DNA is expressed, thereby affecting muscular tone, mood, and energy levels.

It is crucial that before you embark on a series of diets, lifestyle changes, and medication, you should first determine whether genetics is a factor in your health. Effective actions can only be taken after genetic problems have been ruled out as a possibility. If you commit to losing weight and getting healthy, you want to ensure that your efforts are not in vain. You expect to see a return on your investment of time and money in your weight loss journey.

Discoveries are made in the scientific community on a daily basis. For example, according to studies, the majority of people who lose weight on a diet regain the weight they lost, usually within five years. You might be wondering why this is. The answer is straightforward – Hormonal Imbalance. It is vital to maintain hormonal balance in order to accomplish long-term weight loss. Only when your hormones are in balance can you lose weight and keep it off for good.

According to an endocrinologist, hormonal balance is defined as "having all of your hormones in the proper proportions." All of your hormones are intertwined. Therefore, when one is out of balance, it will have a significant impact on the others.

When your hormones are balanced, your general quality of life improves. As a result, you will have a healthy and functional body. You will not experience excessive hunger or cravings, and your metabolism will work to keep your body at a healthy weight. Despite your increased energy, you are unlikely to suffer anxiety or worry. This will have a positive impact on your mood. Your sleep pattern improves, leading to longer and quality sleep that helps relax and repair your body. Hormonal balance is linked to better health and longer life.

Fat Gene

A large number of genes have been identified as being involved in the regulation of body weight, metabolism, hunger, and body fat distribution. In fact, hundreds of genes have been identified as being associated with obesity to date. Because of our genetic composition, our hormonal systems are almost identical to those of our ancestors. Moreover, these have remained unchanged over the course of several generations.

Unfortunately, our environment has changed even while our hormonal systems have remained unchanged over time. Today, many nutritionists believe that we should eat the same way our forefathers did thousands of years ago. However, this is impossible because times have changed. For example, unlike now that there is surplus food production, it was a major issue back then. The ancient tribes of Africa, Mexico, and India ate a high-carbohydrate, whole-grain diet rich in fiber. The result was always the same - a hormonal balance and lean body composition.

Today, however, we are looking for a "one-size-fits-all" solution. That is why there are so many diet books that contradict each other. Obesity is possible in modern times because our civilization's food disrupts the delicate hormonal balance that has been genetically imprinted into our bodies. Various authors select the cuisine of a specific ancient society to match the nutrition they write about in their books. This anthropological basis for dieting falls short because it does not account for hormones.

According to obesity expert George Bray, "genetics is the weapon, the environment is the trigger." Unfortunately, we cannot change our genetic composition for now. We do, however, have the ability to change our hormone levels.

Genes and Weight

For many decades, several researchers have focused their efforts on finding a correlation between genes and the human body. They also attempted to discover how it influences weight gain and regulates the release of fat. The results of one such study revealed a genetic variation that allows energy from food to be retained as fat rather than being burned off as energy. However, despite this study, we cannot ignore the obesity pandemic, which is driven by behavior and environment rather than poor genes.

In a survey on Americans, it was revealed that more than two-thirds of the general public has weight-loss-related issues. For starters, most individuals can already glance down and tell which versions they are most likely to be carrying in their bodies. However, even for younger people, the information may not necessarily be of much assistance.

It is, however, important to note that even after identifying certain genes that might be prevalent in a person, it is important that you don't leave out the influence of environmental and other factors that can contribute to obesity.

Also, having a particular gene may need you to put in more effort to combat the negative consequences associated with it.

Hormones

A lot of people complain that despite restricting their food consumption and engaging in exercise from time to time, they still struggle to lose weight. This may sound impossible following the fact that both exercising and dieting are age-long weight loss techniques. However, it is important to note that there are other factors to consider in situations like this. Therefore, once it is proven that their diets and exercise routine are not the issue, the next thing to consider is their body chemistry, specifically their hormones.

It may appear difficult to lose weight, keep it off, or live a healthy life unless you treat the underlying problem. Therefore, whatever diet, exercise, medication, or thinking you put into it will be in vain unless and until the core source of the problem is addressed – your hormones.

A major component of our obsession with weight is the misunderstood role played by hormones. Yes, losing weight while on a diet is possible, but it doesn't mean you are healthy and may gain it all back again. However, if you follow a healthy, balanced diet high in nutrients, you can achieve long-term weight loss while experiencing little hunger or cravings.

The importance of a healthy diet and regular exercise cannot be ignored. However, there are little messengers within your body called hormones that operate beneath the surface of all of the meal recommendations, exercise programs, and everything else in the dietary dictionary.

Through your hormones, messages are sent and received from the brain to the rest of your body. When we exercise, hormones are released that direct the body to move, consume energy stored to boost certain parts of the body, and shut down others. Also, as soon as you consume a particular food, certain hormones begin to work, informing your body on where the food should go, what effect it will have on your body and your brain, or whether you want to eat more.

Whenever you consume a particular food that upsets your body, whenever you experience depression, pregnancy, or any other kind of emotional, psychological, or physical turmoil - your hormones can malfunction and alter your physical, mental and emotional state.

Also, our metabolism is slowed because of the decline in hormone production that occurs as we grow older.

Hormones and Weight

Whether you are thin or obese, your hormones control your fat cells and fat tissue. It is also important to remember that hormone imbalance does not occur by itself. An intuitive sense that something is wrong with the body exists in many overweight persons. Hormones are responsible for more than just controlling weight; they also influence mood and emotion, appetite, and the body's ability to digest the food that is consumed. The lack of willpower is not the issue here.

Numerous endocrine problems, including excessive cortisol levels in women and low growth hormone and testosterone output in men, are linked to fat storage. These hormonal changes have a significant impact on adipose tissue metabolism and distribution. Thus, hormones, which have powerful interactions with fat cells, significantly influence your weight. Insulin is one of many hormones that are involved in affecting your weight.

Hormones are essential to our existence, and almost all living organisms produce them. These potent chemicals regulate your metabolism. Hormones, for example, determine how much fat you have and where it is stored; they manage your appetite; they affect your energy levels; they influence how you feel, and they even influence your motivation to exercise. Hormones are essential for muscle growth and strengthening. Hormones have an impact on your body weight as well.

Diet and Hormones

When it comes to maintaining a daily routine, diet is the most effective drug. Your diet has the ability to cause or cure illness; every bite you take has an impact on your hormones. In some cases, the sight or smell of food might have an effect on hormone levels.

When we eat, there is a chemical reaction between the food and our hormones. This just further shows that hormones are responsible for regulating the human digestive system. It further controls hunger and cravings, which in turn control your weight.

It is important to note that even though insulin is not the only hormone influenced by diet, it is closely associated with our food consumption.

Hormones in food can sometimes have an effect on us without us even realizing it. This is because substances that mimic hormones are regularly found in the chemicals that are in our food.

Specific meals influence specific hormones. Micronutrients are found in foods and are involved in the regulation of hormone production and processing. Unfortunately, many of the essential nutrients that the body requires for optimal hormone production and efficient hormone function are lacking in today's processed diets. Thyroid hormone and testosterone levels fall as a result of dieting, whereas cortisol (a hormone that stimulates weight gain) rises considerably.

Diets have the potential to destabilize your metabolism. Therefore, it is important to note that when you diet, your metabolism is drastically impacted. In addition, the stress that your body experiences while losing weight might cause all of the hormonal imbalances that cause you to lose interest in sticking with a diet. Dieting, ironically, has the opposite effect of speeding up your metabolism. This is why diet has failed in about 90% of examined cases.

Metabolism

Even though some people have reduced their caloric intake and increased their physical activities, they have failed to lose significant weight. Hence, they blame it on a slow metabolism.

What Is Metabolism?

According to Oxford Learner's Dictionaries, metabolism is defined as "the chemical processes in living things that change food, etc., into energy and materials for growth." Some of these processes include digestion of food, breathing, and conversion of food to energy.

Energy is required for these chemical reactions. The basal metabolic rate, popularly referred to as BMR, refers to the bare minimum of energy your body needs to carry out these chemical reactions. Your BMR can account for up to 80% of your total daily energy requirements, depending on your age and lifestyle.

Does Metabolism Differ?

Your metabolism rate is affected by the following factors: body size, age, gender, and genes.

Because it requires less energy to maintain fat cells than muscle cells, people with more muscle than fat have a faster metabolism.

Fat accumulation and muscle loss are common experiences attached to aging. Therefore, as you grow older, your metabolism rate may slow down.

Men have a faster metabolism than women on average, owing to their higher muscle mass, heavier bones, and lower body fat levels.

To some extent, your genes may influence your metabolism. This is because genes influence your muscle size and growth ability, both of which have an impact on your metabolism.

Metabolism and Weight

Overweight people, according to research, have faster metabolisms than thin people. This is because larger bodies require more energy to perform basic bodily functions.

Another factor could be what you consume after setting aside the possibility of slow metabolism in weight gain. Overeating and drinking are more often than not the causes of weight gain, rather than a slow metabolism. This happens when you consume more calories than you burn.

If you want to lose weight and keep it off, you must track how many calories you consume, even though this may be difficult to accept.

Crash diets and other calorie-restricted diets can cause your metabolism rate to slow down significantly.

When you follow certain diets, your body is forced to break down muscle to obtain enough energy, which slows down your metabolism. When you have less muscle and a slower metabolism, it is much easier to regain the weight you lost while on the diet even after you stop it.

Several foods and beverages have been promoted as having the ability to boost your metabolism. However, there hasn't been scientific proof of it. While you have little control over the rate at which your metabolism works, you may influence how many calories you burn by increasing or decreasing your physical activity level. Remember, the more active you are, the more calories you burn. However, being active doesn't mean that you have a fast metabolism rate.

It only helps you burn calories. Some of the easy and effective ways to burn calories are walking and swimming.

Hormones and Metabolism

The rate at which you burn calories is a crucial factor in determining your weight. For example, if Male A gains weight after consuming the same amount of food and Male B does not, one may begin to wonder why there is a variance between the results. Well, this variance has something to do with metabolism. Those with a fast metabolism will burn off the calories, while those with a slow metabolism will store them in their bodies as fat.

Hormones and metabolic rate contribute mainly to the inconsistency that exists between people who eat a lot but gain no weight and others who limit calories but gain weight.

Fortunately, most of us have a somewhat efficient metabolism. This means that the food you consume is burned effectively, conserving as much energy as possible. However, unlike a machine, the more it works, the less food is needed to keep your metabolism working smoothly. Therefore, when there is leftover food in your system, it is transformed into fat.

Genetics has been discovered to be the reason the majority of us have such a rapid metabolism. This is because we have been genetically selected for our ability to burn fat efficiently.

Some people with slow metabolisms have lived a long time. These are the people who eat and never seem to gain weight. This is because their internal systems are so inefficient; they have to eat as much food as possible to keep their bodies working; as a result, there is never enough left over to be stored as fat. As a result, the metabolically inefficient can consume large amounts of food without becoming overweight. There are numerous ways to boost your metabolism, and enhancing your metabolism will improve your general health.

Having a metabolism that is both efficient and slow can leave you feeling sluggish and exhausted all of the time. When you increase the rate at which your metabolism works, you burn calories more quickly. Unfortunately, there is no perfect remedy that can be used to achieve this goal. The medications that do claim to accomplish this have adverse effects, such as making your heart beat faster or causing other imbalances, which produce psychological and physiological stress on the body and should be avoided and only taken in line with medical advice.

In conclusion, a slow metabolism can be caused by specific medical disorders; however, this is not always the case. If you suspect that you have a problem that isn't responding to lifestyle changes, you should seek medical advice.

CHAPTER 3:
IDENTIFICATION OF BODY TYPE

There are a couple of tests you can do online to help you figure out your body type. Although after going over the characteristics of an ectomorph, Mesomorph, and Endomorph, you should have an indication of what body type you are. There are some questions you may need to answer under the following tests:

- ➤ **The wrist test:** Is there a space between your middle finger and thumb when you try to wrap it over the opposite wrist? If there is, it means you have a larger frame. On the other hand, you have a regular structure if the fingers touch slightly, and if the fingers overlap, you have a small frame.

- ➤ **Bone test:** Do you have noticeable facial bones? Is it possible that your face is delicate and round? Usually, angular faces gravitate toward the more slender forms, whereas endomorphs have rounder, gentler features.

➢ **Shoulder test:** Do your shoulders have a wider range of motion than your hips? If this is the case, you may be a mesomorph or Ectomorph.

➢ **Waist test:** Is your stomach tucked in? If this is the case, you may be a mesomorph.

➢ **Hand and Feet test:** Do your hands and feet appear to be too small or too big for your stature? Endomorphs have small hands and feet, whereas ectomorphs have larger and longer hands and feet.

Do people have more than one body type?

Individuals may notice that they don't always fit clearly into one body type. You may find that you have characteristics from more than one body type, referred to as a mixed / combination /hybrid body type.

➢ **Ecto** - Mesomorph - Lean & Muscular

➢ **Meso** - Endomorph - Strong with less defined muscles

➢ **Endo** - Mesomorph - Skinny-fat / naturally thin but gain weight due to lack of exercise and poor diet.

In research on body types, it was discovered that many people had characteristics of all three body types. Furthermore, the results of the research revealed these proportions of mixed body types:

➢ 3% ecto-mesomorphs

➢ 6.1% (endo-ecto split) mesomorphs

➢ 16.7% meso-endomorphs

➢ 17.1% meso-endomorphs

➢ 51.6% of endo-mesomorphs

Unless you fall under the category of those with an equal mix, it is advisable to stick with what you're most comfortable. Gradually you can switch to a different body type if you discover that a diet plan or workout routine for one body type isn't working for you or if you reach a plateau.

Distinctions between the 3 structural body types

Ectomorphs

These people will perform at their best if they maintain a lean body mass of less than 8-10 percent body fat for men and 12-15 percent for women. Because of their natural composition, they will benefit from training and competing in endurance sports such as triathlons (running, cycling, and swimming), as well as modest strength activities. However, ectomorphs generally struggle when competing as a competitive powerlifter, bodybuilder, or in impact sports with larger persons. There are always significant outliers, but these endeavors are frequently met with disappointment because they are not well adapted to this body type.

Mesomorphs

People with mesomorphic features will perform best if they stay slim, with men keeping 10-15 percent body fat and women maintaining 15-20 percent body fat. They thrive at running, cycling, rowing, swimming, bodybuilding, and impact sports.

People with mesomorphic features do well in most of the typical sports that most people participate in and are frequently referred to as "natural athletes" by others who observe them. However, when people with the mesomorphic feature strive to become overly slim or allow themselves to develop too much body fat, they often struggle.

Endomorphs

People with endomorphic features will perform best if they stay slim for their frame, with men keeping 15-20 percent body fat and women retaining 20-25 percent body fat. They thrive at activities that require strength and size, such as impact sports or less common hobbies like open-water swimming. However, they frequently struggle in sports like bodybuilding, demanding a particular amount of leanness and aesthetics, and activities requiring weight-bearing endurance, such as running.

Female endomorphs are unable to transform into ectomorphs. Regardless of whether you force your body to adapt and shed a significant amount of weight, you will tend to lose muscle. Your goal should always be to make your body the best it can be, not to alter it to something it isn't.

Male endomorphs, on the other hand, prefer to be mesomorphs rather than ectomorphs. This can happen if you put in the time and effort. However, you should continue to strive to be your best self rather than altering your body's form unnaturally.

A typical issue with people who have endomorphic characteristics is that they do not participate in physical conditioning activities on a regular basis, resulting in deconditioning. As a result, they tend to gain considerable body fat while losing muscle mass due to their lack of activity. Obesity and obesity-related disorders such as diabetes and arthritis can affect these individuals, more frequently than their ectomorphic and mesomorphic counterparts.

Can your body type change?

The hereditary characteristics we inherit from our parents contribute to our unique physical appearance. This means that we most likely take after one or both of our parents in relation to our appearance. It's almost impossible to predict what type of body you will have all through the course of your life. A combination of factors such as diet, workout habits, unexpected metabolic changes caused by pregnancy and menopause (for women), injuries, and age can all alter your body type. In addition, your physique may have also changed as a result of lifestyle factors, resulting in you being more of a hybrid body type.

In summary, your body type may change depending on your lifestyle and inherited traits.

Body Measurement

Various body measurements are required to determine your body type. These scores are read from a chart along with your age and gender.

The measurements that are taken are:

> ➢ The size of bones
> ➢ Weight
> ➢ Height
> ➢ Fat
> ➢ Muscle mass

In each of the above categories, a score of 7 will be assigned. Fatness is classified under Endomorph, muscularity is classified under Mesomorph, and thinness is classified under Ectomorph. Once these measurements are confirmed, they can be plotted on a somato chart. For example, if Male B's somatotype measurement is 6:4:2, this implies his fat is 6 out of 7, his muscle is 4 out of 7, and his thinness is 2 out of 7.

Fat Measurement

Men tend to gain fat in their lower bellies as they age, but women accumulate fat in their thighs and buttocks. Thin people feel the cold considerably more than obese ones because fat helps retain heat. Skinfold calipers are used to measure your body fat, or skinfolds, at four different locations on your body to determine your somatotype.

In conclusion, you may achieve maximum results and get into the best shape of your life regardless of your body type if you adapt the appropriate diet with the optimal macronutrient ratios and follow the right workout plan. It's easy to feel envious of others' body types and desire what you don't have. However, you must note that you can live your best life only if you focus on doing what is ideal for your body type.

INTRODUCTION TO HEALTHY DIETING

"When you hear the word "dieting" what is the first thing that comes to your mind?"

While researching this chapter, one of the questions I included in the survey is the one above. I could easily point out a recurring notion in my response from those who participated in the survey. This explains that a large percentage of people in our society have already formed an opinion on dieting, which may not exactly be correct.

A healthy diet doesn't just involve cutting down certain food components or rationalizing food portions. Instead, it is rationalizing food portions in a prescribed way to achieve a specific health goal, and in this case, we will be dealing with weight loss.

One prominent problem that is usually attached to weight-related issues is cardiovascular diseases. Individuals diagnosed with such conditions have restricted themselves from certain foods or drinks that may have been their favorite just to stay alive. However, those that don't fall into that category are striving not to. Hence, the purpose of this chapter.

This chapter will introduce beginners to the science of healthy dieting, and for those who are already on the path, it will expand your knowledge on how to maintain a healthy lifestyle through dieting. The chapter will also clarify some misconceptions about diets and teach the benefits of maintaining a healthy diet.

Furthermore, this chapter will provide a practical recommended meal plan with samples for the different body types as well as options for vegans and non-vegetarians. Also, you will learn about calorie deficit and tracking calories. Hence, you will still be able to enjoy your favorite meals and satisfy your cravings without fear or worry.

In summary, regardless of how complicated or challenging starting a healthy diet may seem, it is a journey that's worth it. Hence, you shouldn't just see it as controlling your food and drink intake but as a lifestyle, an amazing journey to guarantee a long, healthy, and happy life.

Diet Misconceptions

According to Merriam-webster Medical dictionary, diet is defined as "the kind and amount of food prescribed for a person or animal for a specific reason."

Following so many weight loss theories and technological advancements today, many people seek health and nutrition advice from social media rather than professional nutritionists, dietitians, and other health practitioners. Unfortunately, this has led to various circulating misconceptions, which has made so many people confused. Sometimes, one may mistake these misconceptions as professional advice, following how profound they appear and how popular they have become.

Some of these misconceptions include:

Weight loss involves skipping meals

According to a study, this is false. You can't be healthy if you're hungry all day and then end the day with a large meal that compensates for all the calories you skipped earlier. Compared to people who lose weight by consuming fewer calories, those who skip meals lose more muscle than fat.

The study states that those who skip breakfast and eat fewer meals throughout the day are more likely to be overweight than those who eat a nutritious breakfast and eat four or five meals. A logical explanation for this is that persons who miss meals are more likely to feel hungry later on, consuming more calories than they would typically need because they want to be full.

The consumption of several little meals throughout the day may also assist people in controlling their appetite. However, it is advisable to eat small, frequent meals throughout the day consisting of various nutritious foods to keep your energy levels high and your metabolism running smoothly.

Carbohydrates are strictly prohibited:

Today, many diets restrict carbohydrates. However, you should note that it is the primary source of energy for our bodies. The National Health Service (NHS) stated in the United Kingdom that starchy foods should account for one-third of your total calorie intake. Complex carbs, such as those found in brown bread and other wholegrain products, are preferable because they slowly release sugar into the bloodstream, ensuring a steady supply of energy, and they keep you feeling fuller for longer lengths of time. Carbs are highly beneficial when consumed in appropriate quantities.

Diets aren't compulsory when you exercise:

Many people believe that as long as they walk or jog at least thirty minutes a day, they don't have to bother with a healthy diet in their lives. However, this isn't true. For example, Female A walks around the park and then returns home to eat a whole pizza. You will agree that she wasted her time because she will regain the calories she burnt during their walk. If you want to maintain a healthy weight loss plan, you need to understand that a healthy diet and exercise go hand-in-hand. It is advised that you strike a balance between your calorie intake and exercise.

Fats are unhealthy:

Many people feel that adopting a low-fat diet is essential for weight loss even though this misconception is being gradually refuted. It is, however, necessary in sustaining optimal health that we consume enough dietary fat. Also, depriving your body of the essential and required healthy fat will only expose you to health problems. Foods like olives, avocados, almonds, and fatty fish are great for your heart and cholesterol levels, and they are easy to add to any diet. The goal is to ingest a healthy combination of fats in moderation.

Liquids are compulsory for weight loss:

You need to maintain a certain level of hydration; however, excessive intake of high-calorie drinks is harmful. Sodas/fizzy drinks and other high-calorie liquids (beverages like coffee and smoothies can add hundreds of calories to your daily intake. These beverages are not nutritious, and they increase your chances of gaining weight. Therefore, it would be best to consume the volume of liquid equivalent to half your body weight in ounces every day, with water being the most recommended liquid. However, if you cannot consume that much water, you can consume other healthier options like green tea.

Dietary supplements are compulsory:

It's not surprising that more than one-third of Americans take multivitamin and or mineral supplements. It may improve your health in certain ways, such as ensuring adequate intake of underutilized nutrients. However, it may be harmful to others, such as causing you to consume some nutrients in excess to the point that they are toxic to your health.

The focus should remain on what you need by making dietary modifications and, in some instances, taking specific micronutrient supplements, such as vitamin B or vitamin D.

Although we make discoveries every day, there is still a lot we don't know about food components and their interactions with various systems in our bodies, especially since such interactions might vary from person to person. So, until we have a perfect understanding of the human body and its nutritional requirements, it is safer to eat a balanced diet with minimally processed food rather than reliance on meal supplements.

In conclusion, supplements do have a place in our lives. Some people may benefit from supplementing their diet with vitamins or minerals. But, on the other hand, supplements should be used to enhance, not replace, a well-balanced diet.

Introduction To Calories

Following how vital food is to the human body, it is not surprising that there are different notions attached to it, especially for issues connected with weight loss. For example, one of the common statements about weight loss is "you need to consume fewer calories than you burn for you to shed excess fat successfully." Although this is true, and it might be somewhat challenging to estimate your food portion initially, calorie counting makes it a lot easier.

What are calories? According to Cambridge Dictionary, a calorie is "a unit used in measuring the amount of energy food provides when eaten and digested." Generally, it is used to measure the total energy content in foods. The calories we consume are what we use for our daily activities - eating, walking, and essential functions such as breathing. Therefore, consuming more calories than your body needs will lead to excess weight gain.

Factors such as your age, day-to-day level of activity, gender, and weight will determine the number of calories that will be sufficient for you. Therefore, you should note that you can't determine the number of calories you need by comparing yourself to someone else because everyone's body composition is different.

Essentially, to lose weight, you will need to introduce a calorie or caloric deficit. A calorie deficit refers to a state where the body burns more calories than it consumes. This means that you eat fewer calories than your body burns.

Counting Calories

To help you determine your daily calorie intake requirement, it is necessary that you count your calories. This can be determined based on your body composition and lifestyle. Following the advancement of technology, it is much easier to count and track calories. This is because there are numerous websites and online apps that have been specially created for this purpose. However, you can also track or count your calories manually.

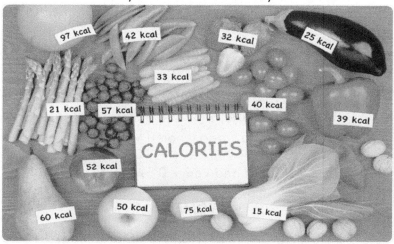

Photo source: *news-medical.net*

There are two things that you need to determine to calculate your calorie requirements manually. They are:

Resting Energy Expenditure [REE]

This refers to the total calories a person burns at rest. This covers calories that you burn when you are asleep or doing absolutely nothing.

Total Daily Energy Experience [TDEE]

This refers to the total calories your body burns in a day. It includes your body's internal and external activities.

REE Formulas

To calculate your REE, follow the formula below.

MEN

[10 x WEIGHT (kg)] + [6.25 x HEIGHT (cm)]
– [5 x age (years)] + 5

OR

[10 x WEIGHT (lbs)] + [6.25 x HEIGHT (Inches)]
– [5 x age (years)] + 5

Note: 1 kg = 2.205 lbs and 1 cm = 0.394 inch

WOMEN

[10 x WEIGHT (kg)] + [6.25 x HEIGHT (cm)]
– [5 x age (years)] – 161

OR

[10 x WEIGHT (lbs)] + [6.25 x HEIGHT (Inches)]
– [5 x age (years)] – 161

Note: 1 kg = 2.205 lbs and 1 cm = 0.394 inch

For practice, let's calculate the REE for:

Male A, who is 32-years old, weighs 85kg and is 135cm tall and Male B, who is 32-years old, weighs 187 lbs and is 53 inches tall.

Female A, who is 23-years old, weighs 50kg and is 126cm tall and Female B, who is 23-years old, weighs 110 lbs and is 50 inches tall.

Male A – [10 x 85] + [6.25 x 135] – [5 x 32] + 5
850 + 843.75 – 160 + 5
= 1538.75

Male B - [10 x 187] + [6.25 x 53] - [5 x 32] + 5
1870 + 331.25 - 160 + 5
= 2046.25

This means that Male A's REE is 1538.75 calories and Male B's REE is 2046.25 calories.

Female A - [10 x 50] + [6.25 x 126] - [5 x 23] - 161
500 + 787.5 - 115 - 161
= 1011.5

Female B - [10 x 110] + [6.25 x 50] - [5 x 23] - 161
1100 + 312.5 - 115 - 161
= 1136.5

This means that Female A's REE is 1011.5 calories and Female B's REE is 1136.5 calories.

TDEE Formulas

To calculate your TDEE, you will multiply your REE by your activity level. Below are different levels of activity.

Sedentary:
x 1.2 [limited exercise]

Lightly active:
x 1.475 [light exercise less than three days a week]

Moderately active:
x 1.55 [moderate exercise five days a week]

Very active:
x 1.725 [hard exercise every day]

Extra active:

x 1.9 [strenuous exercise two or more times a day]

If Male A is moderately active, his TDEE is [1538.75 x 1.55], which is approximately 2,400 calories.

If Male B is moderately active, his TDEE is [2046.25 x 1.55], which is approximately 3,200 calories.

If Female A is moderately active, her TDEE is [1011.5 x 1.55], which is approximately 1,600 calories.

If Female B is moderately active, her TDEE is [1136.5 x 1.55], which is approximately 1,800 calories.

Depending on your specific health goal, calories can either be added or subtracted from your total expenditure. However, to achieve your weight loss goals, you must consume fewer calories than you expend.

Calories and the body

Besides understanding the science behind calories, it is also important to know how it affects you and how the human body uses them. Having established that, you should pay more attention to the food you eat. This is because these calories are absorbed from the components of what you eat or drink. Generally, our meals consist of three macronutrients. They are carbohydrates, proteins, and fats.

Each of these macronutrients has an amount of energy that it supplies the body:

> **Carbohydrate**: 4 calories per gram

> **Protein**: 4 calories per gram
>
> **Fat**: 9 calories per gram

During digestion, the body works on the ingested food by breaking it down into bits. It is these smaller units of food that help the body to carry out the following:

> **Digestion**: Your body will use a certain percentage of the calories you consume to aid the digestion and metabolism of the foods you consume.

> **Basic Funtions**: The energy derived from calories is used to fuel the various body systems to ensure that body parts are functioning properly.

> **Physical Activity**: The body uses calories from the food consumed to fuel your physical activity, which involves exercise and your daily tasks.

Does Counting Calories Work?

Other than being a theory that has stood the test of time, various studies have proven that tracking food intake and counting calories are effective ways to achieve weight loss goals. Some of the reasons calories counting works are:

> **Identification**: It helps you identify the appropriate eating pattern to adopt to achieve your weight loss goals.

> **Awareness**: It creates awareness. It provides the necessary information about your caloric intake and helps you reduce it and track your progress.

> ➢ **Accountability**: It brings about accountability. Tracking your caloric intake helps you to avoid foods that are detrimental to your weight loss target.

However, it is essential to note that not all calories are the same, neither do they have the same effect on your body or overall health. Hence, instead of basing your food menu choices on calories, you should focus more on highly nutritious food.

Introduction To Macronutrients

Counting macronutrients is another popular diet theory. It is a similar concept to calories counting.

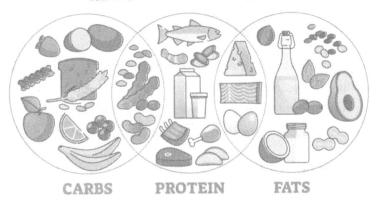

Photo source: _iStock_

What are macronutrients?

This is commonly known as "macros." It refers to the three categories of food nutrients that supply the body with energy. Therefore, when people talk about counting calories, they refer to tracking the grams of carbs, protein, and fat they consume.

Carbohydrates

These are also called "carbs." Carbs include fibers, sugars, and starches found in fruits, beans, grains, vegetables, and dairy products. Carbs are essential for supplying the body with energy. When you eat carbs, the body breaks it down into blood sugar or glucose, which it then uses as fuel or stores as glycogen. Usually, carbs consist of 4 calories per gram. Hence, it makes up the most considerable portion of the caloric intake of a lot of people. Health organizations have recommended that your daily calorie intake from carbs should be between 45 t0 65%.

Protein

Found in fish, eggs, whole grains, and poultry. Protein is essential for bodybuilding, immune functions, cell signaling, and replacing worn-out body tissue. It consists of 4 calories per gram. Although protein recommendations may vary based on certain factors such as age and body composition, the recommended daily calorie intake from protein should be between 10 to 35%.

Fat

Found in nuts, oils, fatty fish, avocado, cheese, and butter. Of all the macronutrients, fats provide the highest calories - 9 calories per gram. Fats are essential for energy and specific functions like maintaining body temperature, hormone production, and nutrient absorption. Health organizations have recommended that your daily calorie intake from fats should be between 20 t0 35%.

Counting Macronutrients

Although this may appear a little challenging for beginners, you'd get better at it with constant practice. The steps involved in counting your macronutrients are:

> ➢ **Know your daily caloric requirement**: The requirements and steps needed to calculate this are stated in the section for calculating calories.

> ➢ **Know your appropriate macronutrient breakdown**: Once you have figured out your daily calorie intake, the next thing to do is to adopt a macronutrient ratio that will work for you.
>
> In order to fit into your specific goals, you may have to alter the recommended intake ratios.

> ➢ **Track your macros**: After choosing an ideal macronutrient ratio, the next step is to track your macros. You can do this by logging in the details online [app or website] or manually [food journal].
>
> Some of the online options provide a digital scale that helps you track your macros. Other options include a barcode scanner that makes it easy to scan the back of a product purchased at a grocery store and gives you the exact macros contained in that particular type of food.

Example of calculating macros

Calculate the macronutrient for a 2000-calorie diet consisting of 35% carbs, 35% protein, and 30% fat.

Carbs

35% of 2000 calories = 700 calories per day

The total amount of carbs allowed per day = Total calories/calories per gram

700/4 = 175 grams
Note: 1 gram = 0.0022 lbs
175 g = 0.4 lbs

Protein

35% of 2000 calories = 700 calories per day

The total amount of protein allowed per day = Total calories/calories per gram

700/4 = 175 grams
Note: 1 gram = 0.0022 lbs
175 g = o.4 lbs

Fat

30% of 2000 calories = 600 calories per day

The total amount of protein allowed per day = Total calories/calories per gram

600/9 = 66.67 grams

Note: 1 gram = 0.0022 lbs

66.67 g = o.15 lbs

From the above example, your daily diet should consist of 175 grams/0.4 pounds of carbs, 175 grams/ 0.4 pounds of protein, and 67 grams/ 0.15 pounds of fat.

Benefits of Counting Macros

➢ **Promotes weight loss**: Since counting macros involves extensive dietary rules, it is effective for weight loss and, sometimes, weight maintenance.

➢ **Increased nutritional value**: By measuring macros, you tend to focus on the nutritional worth of meals rather than calorie intake. This also helps you to make better food selections to meet your macro requirements.

➢ **Helps with specific health goals**: Counting macros is common among people who have health goals. It helps to ensure the consumption of the right macros, which helps achieve specific health goals.

Macros should be set with specific goals in mind, like fat loss or muscle gain. A specific macro-driven diet can be tailored to help achieve these goals.

Basal Metabolic Rate (BMR)

The number of calories a person burns while their body performs its core functions is known as their Basal

Metabolic Rate (BMR). On the other hand, the calories expended when the body is at rest are referred to as the Resting Metabolic Rate (RMR). The BMR is commonly used to determine how fast a person's body burns calories.

It is important to determine your BMR as it accounts for about 70% of the total calories you burn. It includes the energy your body expends to maintain its essential functions - digestion, circulation, respiration, and cell production. Factors such as age, height, weight, food, environment, and gender can influence your BMR.

BMR Formula

Other than the various online apps and websites that we can use to calculate your BMR, you can also calculate it manually using the formulas below. However, it is essential to provide your height, weight, age, and gender to get an accurate answer. The Harris-Benedict equation is commonly used to calculate BMR.

MEN

88.362 + [13.397 x WEIGHT (kg)] +
[4.799 x HEIGHT (cm)] - [5.677 x AGE (years)]

OR

88.362 + [13.397 x WEIGHT (lbs)] +
[4.799 x HEIGHT (inches)] - [5.677 x AGE (years)]

Note: 1 kg = 2.205 lbs and 1 cm = 0.394 inch

WOMEN

447.593 + [9.247 x WEIGHT (kg)] +
[3.098 x HEIGHT (cm)] – [4.330 x AGE (years)]

OR

447.593 + [9.247 x WEIGHT (lbs)] +
[3.098 x HEIGHT (inches)] – [4.330 x AGE (years)]

Note: 1 kg = 2.205 lbs and 1 cm = 0.394 inch

EXAMPLE

1. Calculate the BMR of Male A, who is 34-years old, weighs 83kg and is 185cm tall, and Male B, who is 34-years old, weighs 184 lbs and is 73 inches tall.

Male A

88.362 + [13.397 x 83] + [4.799 x 185] – [5.677 x 34]
88.362 + 1111.951 + 887.815 – 193.018
= 1895.11

Male B

88.362 + [13.397 x 184] + [4.799 x 73] – [5.677 x 34]
88.362 + 2465.048 + 350.327 – 193.018
= 2710.719

Male A has a BMR of approximately 1,900 calories from the above calculations, and Male B has a BMR of approximately 2,700 calories.

1. Calculate the BMR of Female A, who is 34-years old, weighs 77kg and is 152cm tall, and Female B, who is 34-years old, weighs 170lbs and is 60 inches tall.

Female A

447.593 + [9.247 x 77] + [3.098 x 152] - [4.330 x34]
447.593 + 712.019 + 470.896 - 147.22
= 1483.288

Female B

447.593 + [9.247 x 170] + [3.098 x 60] - [4.330 x 34]
447,593 + 1571.99 + 185.88 - 147.22
= 2058.243

From the above calculations, Female A has a BMR of approximately 1,500 calories, and Female B has a BMR of roughly 2,100 calories.

Shopping Guide

A weight-loss diet is flexible and may vary from one person to the other depending on personal preferences. However, there are some necessary ingredients that you must include in your grocery list when you are about to start a healthy diet. Hence, this section will be divided into two to fit both non-vegetarians (those who consume meat) and vegetarians.

Non-Vegetarians

➢ **Meat**: Meats are usually heavy in protein; hence, they can be classified as weight-loss friendly. This is because a diet with high protein can increase your daily calorie expenditure by over eighty calories. Examples are chicken, beef, pork, and turkey.

➢ **Seafood**: A source of protein that helps in building and repairing tissue and helps complement exercise, which makes weight loss achievable. Examples are salmon, shellfish, shrimp, cod, etc.

➢ **Eggs**: A great source of protein that can be enjoyed in a variety of ways.

➢ **Vegetables**: Besides being a healthy, tasty, and colorful addition to meals, vegetables also help regulate blood sugar since they are rich in fiber. The fiber and water in vegetables are easily absorbed. They are a great addition to meals as they are low in calories and can be consumed in higher volumes which helps with weight maintenance. Examples are onions, kale, carrots, broccoli, and peppers.

➢ **Fruits**: Fruits are highly nutritional and serve multiple purposes. They are a significant source of vitamins. Examples are oranges, strawberries, apples, avocados, bananas, etc.

➢ **Tubers**: Tubers contain a high amount of carbohydrates and fibers. It is a suitable recommendation for those on a weight loss diet plan. Examples are yams and potatoes.

➢ **Nuts and Seeds**: These contain a high amount of fiber and protein. They also contain healthy fats, which is an essential requirement for the body. Examples are walnuts, almonds, pumpkin seeds, hazelnuts, etc.

➢ **Healthy Fats and Oil**: Healthy fats and oils are essential to the body to help it fight heart diseases. Examples are coconut oil, extra virgin olive oil, avocado oil, etc.

➢ **Herbs and Spices**: This helps reduce the risk of diabetes and is an excellent way of enhancing your recipes by providing aroma and taste to meals. This includes garlic, salt, turmeric, etc.

➢ **Dairy Products**: Dairy products are rich in vitamins, proteins, and minerals. They are essential in protecting the body and also helping to fight against diseases. Examples are yogurt, milk, cheese, etc.

Vegetarians

➢ **Protein**: Lean proteins are highly recommended for vegetarians. They include yogurt, cheese, tofu, eggs, tempeh, nuts, chickpeas, milk (dairy or non-dairy), etc.

➢ **Healthy Fats**: Healthy fats are essential for metabolism as they help you control your appetite and avoid overeating. Adding monounsaturated fats to your diet will build up your body to fight diseases. Examples are avocado, nut butter, coconut oil, and olive oil.

➢ **Nuts and Seeds**: These contain fiber and protein. It has been proven that people stay for long hours after eating them without getting hungry. Examples are chia seeds, lentils, walnuts, cashews, almonds, dried fruits, etc.

➢ **Vegetables**: This is the primary food group for vegetarians. Adding vegetables to your diet helps with weight loss. They contain essential nutrients for enhancing overall good health. Examples are kale, tomatoes, bell peppers, zucchini, spinach, etc.

➢ **Herbs and Spices**: Spices help to boost metabolism. Examples are salt, chili powder, garlic, oregano, black pepper, etc.

➢ **Frozen Food**: These could be frozen vegetables - edamame, peas, corn, green beans, etc. or frozen fruits - pineapple, berries, mango, etc. Usually, eating vegetables and fruits helps to maintain weight. However, several studies have shown that adults who eat more frozen fruits and vegetables have a lower BMI than those who don't.

➢ **Fruits**: Fruits contain lower calories and more fiber which makes them an essential option for weight loss. Examples are bananas, apples, berries, grapes, oranges, etc.

➢ **Liquids**: You must stay hydrated at all times during your diet. Therefore, some recommendations apart from water are coconut water, green tea, black coffee, and naturally flavored seltzer.

Healthy Diet for Different Body Types

Once you've identified and understood your body type, the next thing is to figure out which diet plan is suitable for you. Just as the three structural body types are different in appearance, diet plans will also vary accordingly.

Weight loss isn't just about eating healthy and exercising, as most people think. If it were, people on a diet would not be complaining about not losing weight even after adopting a diet plan and exercising. Different researchers have proven that your body type reveals information. Some of this information includes how much muscle or fat you have and your metabolism rate. These two factors have a significant impact on your weight loss journey. Although you can have a mix of two body types, according to Catudal, identifying your dominant body will help you develop healthy habits and set more realistic goals. For example, it is illogical for a person with a mesomorph body type to expect the same results as an endomorph even if they eat the same thing. In other words, this information will help you determine the appropriate diet that will fit your health goals.

Often healthy diet recommendations are nutrient-dense sources of carbs, protein, and healthy fats that are substantial and are consistent across all three diets tested. The most significant distinction between them is their macronutrient ratios, with some foods being more suited to specific body types than others. An endomorph, for example, would eat a high-protein breakfast, such as eggs rather than oatmeal, because traditional wisdom holds that this body type benefits from having fewer carbohydrates.

Endomorph

Did you ever make a plan to cut down your food consumption and realize that you barely made it through the first day? Well, numerous studies have shown that this is a common problem among endomorphs. This is because one feature of endomorphs is an intense desire for food which makes it hard to regulate food intake. Hence, they are prone to store fat which is often hard to lose.

It is vital to maintain a calorie deficit throughout the day to lose weight as an endomorph. This will include keeping an eye on your macros. Endomorph nutrition should be considered a way of life rather than a diet. The most efficient method to attain long-term success is to incorporate healthy practices into your everyday routine.

Endomorphs have higher body fat percentages than the other body types and are more sensitive to carbs and insulin. As a result, they require a diet with an evenly distributed macronutrient profile of 40-45% protein, 30-40% fat, and 20-30% carbs. Carbohydrates, on the other hand, should be obtained from vegetables and unprocessed, high-fiber starches.

The ideal diet should be low in carbohydrates, no junk food, and lots of vegetables. Hence, the Paleo and Keto diets have been shown to be excellent for endomorphs since each meal has a combination of protein, veggies, and healthy fats. Endomorphs can also benefit from a high-protein meal in the morning to keep their metabolism intact.

Of all the body types, endomorphs are known to have the most difficulty maintaining their physical fitness. This is more due to their high level of body fat and slow digestion rate rather than laziness. One of the major reasons endomorphs are prone to gain fat is because they have difficulty digesting carbs. Hence, carbs ingested are converted to fat before their body can use it as energy. To determine how many calories or macronutrients you should consume, calculating your basal metabolic rate (BMR) and total daily energy expenditure (TDEE) is an effective tool.

Recommended food options are eggs, lean proteins [beef and chicken], fish [trout, salmon], avocadoes, coconut oil, nuts and seeds, vegetables, barley, and potatoes. The number of calories ingested should be 500 to 700 fewer than the number of calories expended daily.

Sample Meal Plan

This section contains a 7-days meal plan sample option to help endomorphs with their healthy diet.

Day 1

BREAKFAST:	Greek yogurt smoothie	214.3 calories
LUNCH:	Brown rice stir-fry with chicken and peppers	387.7 calories
DINNER:	Sweet potato chili	250 calories
SNACKS:	Carrots dipped in peanut butter	216 calories
	Total Calories	1,068 calories

Day 2

BREAKFAST:	Greek yogurt layered with cinnamon, apples, and walnuts	145 calories
LUNCH:	Shrimp stir-fry with bell pepper and broccoli	271 calories
DINNER:	Vegetables and bean soup with grilled chicken breast	286 calories
SNACKS:	Protein shake	360 calories
	Total Calories	1,062 calories

Day 3

BREAKFAST:	Cottage cheese with almonds and cinnamon	249.8 calories
LUNCH:	Kale salad with cucumbers, salmon, and bell peppers	274 calories
DINNER:	Cauliflower rice with shrimp and veggie kabobs	309.4 calories
SNACKS:	Protein bar	200 calories
TOTAL CALORIES		1,033.2 calories

Day 4

BREAKFAST:	Omelet made with peppers and spinach, topped with avocado slices	310 calories
LUNCH:	Avocado tuna and chickpeas salad	345 calories
DINNER:	Turkey tacos lettuce wraps with a slice of avocado	235 calories
SNACKS:	Greek yogurt with sliced almonds	178 calories
Total Calories		1068 calories

Day 5

BREAKFAST:	Egg frittata with tomatoes, onions, and spinach	190 calories
LUNCH:	Brown rice stir fry	139 calories
DINNER:	Salmon steamed broccoli and sautéed mushrooms	306 calories
SNACKS:	Boiled egg and sliced avocado	295 calories
	Total Calories	930 calories

Day 6

BREAKFAST:	Mixed vegetable omelet with slices of avocado	293 calories
LUNCH:	Grilled chicken salad with garbanzo beans, tomatoes, and tzatziki sauce	258 calories
DINNER:	Spiced steak stir-fry with cauliflower rice	355.1 calories
SNACKS:	Hummus and sliced vegetables	90 calories
	Total Calories	996.1 calories

Day 7

BREAKFAST:	Eggs and spinach	313 calories
LUNCH:	Quinoa mixed with cubed chicken breast and chopped vegetables	445.3 calories
DINNER:	Red beans and quinoa soup	223 calories
SNACKS:	Sliced apple with peanut butter	160 calories
Total Calories		1141.3 calories

In summary, slow digestion is associated with a slow metabolism. Therefore, you need to increase the quantity of fibre in your diet to improve digestion. Make an effort to consume foods high in insoluble fibre, such as beans and berries. Lentils, legumes, whole grains are also good options.

Endomorph metabolism is slower than mesomorphs and ectomorphs; therefore, replenishment after exercise is less important than the other two body types. When sweating profusely during an intense workout, consuming a post-workout protein smoothie or a drink may be tempting, but you should choose the lowest calorie options available. Likewise, you should avoid sports drinks with a lot of sugar and sodium.

If you want to eat after your exercise, you should opt for something light. You should also avoid eating 'junk food' related to snacks and carbs. Instead, consume three to four small meals throughout the day, with carbs accounting for the smallest percentage of total calories.

Ectomorph

Do you feel frustrated when you realize that regardless of how much you eat and the number of times you eat in a day, your weight remains the same, and you still appear lanky? From several studies, it has been revealed that it is a common problem prone to ectomorphs. They don't expend many calories, and they struggle to build muscle when needed.

Ectomorphs are thin and slender by nature. As a result, gaining weight or building muscle mass appears to be a difficult task. On the other hand, people with this body type do not have to worry about losing weight because of how their bodies are built. This, however, should not be used as an excuse to disregard nutritional requirements.

The reason ectomorphs find it hard to gain weight can be linked to their fast metabolic rate. Ectomorphs have the most rapid metabolic rate among the different body types. Therefore, following the recommended macronutrient ratio, ectomorphs who wish to grow muscle should consume more protein, carbohydrates, and fewer fats depending on their body fat percentage and exercise routine.

The recommended food for an ectomorph is starchy carbohydrates such as yams and potatoes, brown rice, fruits such as pineapple, avocado, mangoes, peaches, mangoes, pineapple, unsaturated fats -coconut oil and avocado oil, nuts and seeds - sunflower seed butter, nuts, and nut butter, and lean proteins.

For you to ensure that you are getting the required calories for your weight, it is essential to track your calories. As mentioned earlier, you can either do this online or manually. To know the number of calories you need, you should add 200 to 300 calories to your TDEE and BMR. For instance, an ectomorph whose TDEE is 2700 calories will need about 3000 calories to gain a substantial amount of weight.

Naturally, consuming that amount of calories every day can make you feel bloated. However, to avoid that, it is advised that you choose calorie-dense food options that you will eat on a regular basis. Also, you should include snacks in your diet while distributing your required calories between 4 to 6 meals every day.

Another way to increase your calorie intake is by introducing a high-quality protein supplement. For example, if you don't like drinking shakes, you can put whey protein powder into other foods, including smoothies, oatmeal, yogurt, pancake mix, and peanut butter.

Weight gain supplements are incredibly high in sugar, calories, and artificial fillers, which have an adverse effect on your weight and overall health. Therefore, you should avoid them to stay healthy.

Supplements

It is frustrating when you realize that you tend to lose weight easily but take forever to gain weight even after eating the same meals and engaging in the same physical activities as those who can easily gain weight and maintain it. It is even more frustrating when you can't seem to figure out the exact reason for this. A study has revealed that this is an experience that is common to most child ectomorphs. However, as they grow older, they begin to educate themselves by asking questions and through research. Other than the usual healthy dieting and exercise recommendations, experts recommend supplements to ectomorphs to enhance weight and muscle gain. This is because they are "hard gainers." They would require more than the usual recommendations to make any substantial difference in their appearance or achieve their fitness goals.

Despite the various supplement recommendations on the internet today, Creatine Monohydrate has significantly increased muscle mass. Therefore, to ensure that this works effectively, it is essential to increase your insulin level by including food and protein powders in this supplement. Combining regular exercise, a healthy diet consisting of high-quality food, and a supplement [optional] is a key to achieving your desired body.

Sample Meal Plan

This section contains a 7-days meal plan sample option to help ectomorphs with their healthy diet.

Day 1

BREAKFAST:	Sweet potato toast and nut butter	82 calories
LUNCH:	Mediterranean salad with chopped vegetables	230 calories
DINNER:	Whole-grain tortillas and steak fajitas	700 calories
SNACKS:	Protein bar	200 calories
Total Calories		1,212 calories

Day 2

BREAKFAST:	Oatmeal with strawberry and walnut toppings	258 calories
LUNCH:	Turkey chili and salad	251 calories
DINNER:	Brown rice with chicken and mushroom stir-fry	380 calories
SNACKS:	A handful of dried nuts and seeds	108 calories
Total Calories		997 calories

Day 3

BREAKFAST:	Baked sweet potatoes	204 calories
LUNCH:	Turkey sandwich, mashed avocado, and wholegrain bread	395 calories
DINNER:	Avocado and wholegrain crackers	121 calories
SNACKS:	Banana and berry smoothie	318 calories
	Total Calories	1,038 calories

Day 4

BREAKFAST:	Fruit smoothie with protein powder and almond milk	187 calories
LUNCH:	Stir-fry vegetables	256 calories
DINNER:	Grilled chicken, tomato, sautéed kale, and cucumber salad	396 calories
SNACKS:	Carrot and black bean dip	115 calories
	Total Calories	954 calories

Day 5

BREAKFAST:	Low-fat Greek yogurt and wholegrain toast	183 calories
LUNCH:	Avocado toast with fried eggs and salad	247 calories
DINNER:	Turkey and mango tacos with black beans	308.9 calories
SNACKS:	Almonds and apple cake	342 calories
Total Calories		1089 calories

Day 6

BREAKFAST:	Baked quinoa with tomato sauce, vegetables, and chicken	336 calories
LUNCH:	Bean and vegetable burger	198.4 calories
DINNER:	Baked sweet potato	204 calories
SNACKS:	A plate of sliced fruits	200 calories
Total Calories		938.4 calories

Day 7

BREAKFAST:	Vegetable frittata with sweet potatoes	351 calories
LUNCH:	Roasted turkey and vegetables	231 calories
DINNER:	Grilled shrimp and vegetable kabobs with quinoa	353 calories
SNACKS:	Apple and a slice of cheese	266.9 calories
	Total Calories	1201.9 calories

You can increase your calorie intake considerably by consuming 400-500 calorie meals every two to four hours or multiple times a day. Almonds, peanut butter, and apple slices are good recommendations of what you can eat without feeling bloated or full.

Mesomorph

Do you know that having a fit body does not signify good health? Well, a lot of people, including mesomorphs, have failed to realize that health conditions are not restricted to a specific body type. Hence, mesomorphs can be suffering from conditions like diabetes, high blood pressure, and other heart-related diseases and not know because, with their body type, it is assumed that they are healthy.

Therefore, this boils down to the essentials of maintaining a healthy diet.

Since mesomorphs can gain or lose weight easily, it is advised that they opt for a balanced diet. This means that there should be an even distribution of their macronutrients. As we all know, the muscles in the body weigh more than fat, and as such, it requires more calories to maintain. Therefore, mesomorphs need a diet that consists of lean protein and complex carbohydrates. This is because they have a higher muscle mass ratio than the other body types, and they tend to respond better to a diet with high protein. Also, a high-protein diet is recommended to help build, repair, and replace muscles.

Mesomorphs' food recommendations include beans, nuts, butter, greek yogurt, eggs, legumes, pea protein, whole grains, and lentils. Vegetables and fruits (citrus fruits and berries) are rich in vitamins and fiber; therefore, they are recommended to help the body function effectively. Healthy fats too should be included in a mesomorph diet.

Sample Meal Plan

This section contains a 7-days meal plan sample option to help mesomorphs with their healthy diet.

Day 1

BREAKFAST:	Roasted lentils	178 calories
LUNCH:	Pizza with vegetable toppings	440 calories
DINNER:	Tuna niçoise salad	332 calories
SNACKS:	Protein bar	200 calories
	Total Calories	1,150 calories

Day 2

BREAKFAST:	Vegetable frittata and fruits	162 calories
LUNCH:	Vegetable salad and potatoes	176 calories
DINNER:	Spaghetti and tomato sauce	443 calories
SNACKS:	Chocolate protein shake	267 calories
	Total Calories	1048 calories

Day 3

BREAKFAST:	Fruit smoothie with soy milk	106 calories
LUNCH:	Squashed noodles and turkey sauce	290 calories
DINNER:	Brown rice with vegetable stir-fry	197 calories
SNACKS:	Trail mix	462 calories
Total Calories		1,055 calories

Day 4

BREAKFAST:	Greek yogurt parfait	180 calories
LUNCH:	Turkey chili and potatoes	413 calories
DINNER:	Baked salmon and roasted broccoli	384 calories
SNACKS:	Cheese and fruit stick	56 calories
Total Calories		1033 calories

Day 5

BREAKFAST:	Toast and scrambled eggs	263 calories
LUNCH:	Chicken salad	48 calories
DINNER:	Sliced steaks garnished with onions and avocado	323 calories
SNACKS:	A plate of sliced fruits	200 calories
	Total Calories	834 calories

Day 6

BREAKFAST:	Quinoa and vegetables	279.6 calories
LUNCH:	Sweet potato and sautéed kale	233 calories
DINNER:	Vegetable salad	176 calories
SNACKS:	Celery and peanut butter	134 calories
	Total Calories	822.6 calories

Day 7

BREAKFAST:	Almond butter toast with egg	243 calories
LUNCH:	Grilled salmon salad	260 calories
DINNER:	Roasted vegetable and sweet potatoes	210 calories
SNACKS:	Hummus and bell pepper sticks	134 calories
Total Calories		847 calories

When adopting a mesomorph diet, you should remember that your main goal should be maintaining a balance as it is very easy to sway to one side since weight loss and weight gain are easy compared to the other body types.

Food To Avoid

Foods that are highly concentrated in carbs are responsible for releasing sugar into the bloodstream at a rapid rate. Since the body is likely to convert this sugar to fat rather than burn it as energy, it causes a spike in blood sugar level. Also, an Endomorphic body is expected to convert calories extracted from meals into fat. Hence, endomorphs must eliminate dense carbs and calorie-dense meals from their diet. Examples of this calorie-dense and dense carb food to limit as an endomorph are: red meats, alcohol, white bread, highly processed foods, drinks [such as sports drinks, energy drinks, and soft drinks], bagels, high sodium-rich meals, cakes, pasta, chocolate and candy, refined cereal, saturated oil, and rich dairy products.

The primary aim of an ectomorph is to gain weight or muscle mass. Hence, to achieve these goals, it is important to stay away from meals that have low-calorie density. Low-calorie density meals refer to meals that have to be eaten in large quantities or proportions to gain significant weight. Also, since the body burns carbs as energy, limiting highly processed carbohydrates is recommended. Examples of foods to limit as an ectomorph are: chips, soda, candy, popcorn, and lean meat.

Since a mesomorph body type primarily entails striking a balance with meals and physical activities to maintain their body type, there isn't so much regulation. However, to avoid overlap, it is essential to limit or even stay away from foods commonly known to consist of hidden sugars. Such foods include flavored yogurt, cereal bars, ketchup, soft drinks, and beverages.

In conclusion, you would agree that knowing your body type is essential for your diet. It would help you decide the best food options necessary to fuel your body, boost your metabolism, and boost your body's optimal performance. Also, it would help you avoid extreme diets that are not beneficial or, at worst, harmful to your body. For instance, as an ectomorph, you know that you must avoid a low-carb diet like a ketogenic diet because it is detrimental to you. So, instead, your primary diet would be high in carbs. On the other hand, an endomorph whose primary problem is losing weight would opt for a low-carb diet which is beneficial to them.

Remember that the focus is improving your overall health through healthy dieting and not just trying out foods to find a "perfect" diet.

CHAPTER 4:
INTRODUCTION TO EXERCISING

Walking into the gym for the first time would most likely stir up a different feeling in you. This is because, unlike the books you have read or the movies you've watched where almost everyone at the gym would most likely have a defined body, the reverse is the case in reality. Looking around the room filled with different people, you would realize that there are people of different shapes and body types at the gym. But, most importantly, they are there for various reasons.

A common response people who seem to have issues with their physical appearance get when they seek advice from friends, social media, or even health practitioners is "hit the gym." As easy as exercising may sound, there is more to it.

According to the Oxford Dictionary, Exercise is defined as an "activity requiring physical effort, carried out to sustain or improve health and fitness." Therefore, it can also be regarded as a component of physical activities. From this definition, it is proven that exercising is beneficial to the human body.

Benefits Of Exercising

Engaging in exercise is beneficial to both our physical and mental health. Some of these benefits include:

➢ **Weight Loss**: Several studies have shown that one of the major factors responsible for excess weight gain is inactivity. Hence, regular exercise is a recommended activity to counter obesity. Also, since weight loss is mainly dependent on how many calories you burn, it is essential to engage in exercise. This is because regular exercises have been shown to increase the metabolic rate of the body. Furthermore, for people who have already attained a desirable weight, regular exercise will help to maintain muscle mass and weight.

➢ **Reduced Risk Of Chronic Diseases**: In recent times, "chronic diseases" have taken a top spot in the list of causes of death. Chronic diseases like heart diseases and diabetes can be caused by an accumulation of excess belly fat which may result from a lack of activity. However, since studies have shown that regular exercise is a means to improve heart health and insulin sensitivity, regular exercise is recommended to help reduce the risk of these chronic diseases.

➢ **Increased Strength**: Exercise is crucial when it comes to building and maintaining strong muscles and bone density. For example, pairing weightlifting with sufficient protein intake encourages muscle growth. Loss of muscle mass is one of the characteristics of aging, and in order to reduce this, it is important to engage in exercise that helps in promoting your muscle's ability to absorb amino acids.

➤ **Endurance**: Engaging in exercise at least twice a week will help stimulate the endurance and strength of skeletal muscles. This stimulation is beneficial to the body as it improves the flow of blood to the muscles.

➤ **Increased Energy Level**: Exercise has been proven to significantly increase the energy level of people who have Chronic Fatigue Syndrome and other health conditions such as cancer.

➤ **Improved Skin Health**: Engaging in regular and moderate exercise helps to protect the skin cells from oxidative damage. At the same time, exercise helps delay signs of aging as it promotes blood flow to the skin cells.

➤ **Improved Sleep Quality**: According to research, regular exercising can enhance sleep quality and reduce sleep latency, especially in people who have insomnia. In addition, regular exercise can improve deep/REM sleep at night and help you feel energetic during the day. This is because medical studies have revealed that exercising is one of the ways to release endorphins. Endorphins can be described as natural chemicals that help the body deal with stress, pain, depression and trigger feelings of well-being.

➢ **Improved Brain Health and Memory:** Exercise is known to help increase heart rate, which in the long run promotes the flow of blood to the different parts of the body and brain. Also, it enhances the production of hormones which protects the memory and improves thinking and brain function. In summary, regular exercise improves thinking skills, mental function, and overall brain health in both adults and children.

In conclusion, regardless of the type of exercise you engage in, you will notice an inevitable improvement in your mood, physical appearance, mental health, and other aspects of your health once you start engaging in regular exercise.

Principles Of Exercising

Following the introduction to exercise and its benefits, it is important to mention that there are certain principles that you must apply to your exercise plans to ensure that you achieve your fitness goals. The principles in this section were developed from diverse research on fitness and exercise.

1. **Specificity**: Before you begin your exercise plan, the first thing to do is identify your goals. Once this is completed, you then should find exercises in line with such goals. There must be some specificity to

the type of exercise you have adopted to effect change in the human body. This simply means, if your fitness goal is to lose weight, you must train your body to work in line with that goal by adopting exercises that will guarantee weight loss.

2. **Progressive Overload**: Just as the name implies, this principle relies on a progressive increase in your body's demands to achieve your goals. For example, there should be a progressive increase in the weight you lift during your weight training to build muscle mass.

3. **Progression**: Male A wakes up to the news of his friend Male B diagnosed with type 2 diabetes resulting from obesity. Due to fear, Male A goes ahead, signs up in a gym, and begins rigorous training. After the second day at the gym, he can barely move his arms and legs due to muscle fatigue. This illustration reveals a common mistake that we make when exercising. Before you start an exercise program or move to a higher intensity of exercise, you must move at a reasonable rate applicable to your body. There are no set rules or guidelines on this aspect. The rule here is simply to listen to your body and work within its capabilities.

4. **Exercise Intensity**: This principle is a very important one, although many people ignore it. The body undergoes different changes during an exercise session, such as increased metabolic demands, increased heart rate, increased blood

flow, etc. Therefore, before you begin your workout, you must start with a warm-up. Warm-ups are essential as they help the different parts of the body adjust in anticipation of the workout. Also, it is vital to end an exercise session by stretching or warming down. This is because an abrupt cessation of exercise can cause a rapid lowering of blood pressure, leading to fainting, excess blood pump to the parts of the body, or cardiorespiratory complications.

5. **Intensity and Frequency**: Physiologists have debunked the myth that exercises always have to be painful to ensure that you are performing them well. They have advised that exercise intensity should depend on your heart rate and how comfortable you are when exercising. Also, research has shown that exercises should be done at least three to five times a week. This is to ensure consistency in achieving and maintaining your fitness goals. However, you can go beyond this guideline as long as you ensure that you're not over-exercising, leading to stress injuries.

6. **Overall conditioning**: This principle implies that you should ensure a holistic approach to achieve maximum effect on the muscle group and body when adopting a specified plan. This approach should include; increased strength, endurance, flexibility, and maintenance.

Effective application of these principles will ensure that you have an efficient exercise session and achieve your fitness goals in the long run.

Exercise Specific To Your Body Type

Female A and Female B agreed to sign up at a gym. Their reason for signing up was to achieve a lean and toned body. However, after the first session with their instructor, Female A wanted to opt-out because she found the exercises too hard. On the other hand, Female B found the workout easy and was anticipating their next session.

From the above scenario, we can point out that two people can start an exercise program simultaneously, follow all the principles of exercising, and still have different opinions about it. Sometimes, this opinion that they form will determine the result of their session. However, this may largely depend on their body type.

Research on body types has shown that people differ in both psychological and physical adaptations of exercise. This is primarily because their choice of exercise plan will mostly depend on their body composition and type. For example, Male A may enjoy long-term workouts while Male B may not. As a result, Male A will most likely do well in running while Male B will do better in yoga.

There is no universal or perfect exercise. Therefore, each person should adopt an exercise plan that best fits their fitness goal and body type.

Endomorph

Since the primary goal of an endomorph is weight loss and cardiorespiratory improvement, when it comes to exercises, your focus should be on exercises that focus on this aspect. It is recommended that you focus on this even after achieving cardiorespiratory efficiency and your desired body. This is to maintain your weight and ensure you do not regain fat. Experts also advise that you should commit to a lifestyle that is less sedentary. For exercise sessions, your primary focus should be maintaining metabolic conditioning. Other effective strategies for increasing fitness are plyometrics, circuits of resistance exercises, and short rest intervals.

It is no surprise that endomorphs have a slow metabolism and excess body fat. Therefore, their exercise techniques should involve high-intensity exercise routines that focus on aerobic and strength training activities to maximize weight loss while encouraging lean muscle growth. In addition, these exercises are beneficial in increasing the body's daily energy requirement and metabolic efficiency.

An important point to establish is that it is essential to note your total daily calories needed and limit unnecessary food intake while exercising. However, it is more important to include ample protein in every meal to keep the body in a modest negative energy balance with as minimal muscle catabolism as possible. Engaging in daily exercise is an essential tool for endomorphs to achieve their fitness goals.

Besides your regular exercise, it is essential to incorporate weight training into your daily routine. The primary focus of this weight training should be on reducing body fat while increasing metabolic rate and building lean muscle mass.

Exercise Tips

Here are some tips to help you set up an efficient workout plan:

> - **High Reps**: The word 'reps' is a shortened word for repetition. It refers to the number of repetitive movements you perform of the same exercise. A high range of reps will stimulate the muscle and enhance muscle growth at a faster rate. Therefore, incorporating a high rep range of eight to twelve reps is recommended alongside aerobic training.

> - **Circuit Training** involves doing exercises in succession with short breaks of 15 to 60 seconds between each set. Circuit training has been proven to be very effective in weight loss.

> - **Muscle Groups:** Working on larger muscle groups (the chest, legs, back, and shoulders) during an exercise session is effective in weight loss. Hence, it is recommended to concentrate on large muscle groups during workouts.

Following the above resistance tips will assist you in developing a leaner and toned body.

Strength and weight training exercises are vital in practically every weight loss plan, especially for people with an endomorph body type.

Cardiovascular exercises such as running are crucial for endomorphs as it assists in losing weight by burning a large number of calories to create a calorie deficit. In essence, this means that a person is losing weight due to burning more calories than they are consuming.

There are numerous examples of cardiovascular exercises. Some of them include:

High Intensity Interval Training [HIIT]: This is a type of exercise in which a person alternates between a period of very high-intensity exercise and a period of rest or a lower-intensity exercise. It usually lasts for a short time [20 to 30 minutes]. It is recommended for an endomorph to engage in HIIT two to three times weekly to maintain a healthy weight. It is also recommended that they include steady-state cardio of about thirty minutes to one hour.

Slow and Steady State Training [SST]: This type of cardiovascular exercise consists of regular moderate to low-intensity exercises. Usually, these exercises last for a more extended period. Recommended SST exercises for endomorphs include swimming, walking, and jogging for about thirty minutes to one hour, two to three times weekly.

The typical exercise recommendation for endomorphs is compound exercises. Compound exercises refer to the kind of exercises that help you have more control over your body.

Engaging in compound exercises usually involves combining different exercises to reach a target.

Examples of compound exercises are:

- ➤ Bench Press
- ➤ Squats - weighted
- ➤ Deadlift

Sample Exercise Plan

This section consists of a 7-days exercise plan for endomorphs. These exercises are a combination of circuit and resistance training which will help build muscle and, at the same time, enhance fat loss.

Day 1: Resistance Training for Upper Body

WARM-UP
Skipping /jogging for 3-6 minutes

BENCH PRESS
Recommended sets: 4 sets
Reps: 8 -10 reps

SKULL CRUSHERS
Recommended sets: 2 sets
Reps: 10 15 reps

CABLE ROWS
Recommended sets: 3 sets
Reps: 10 12 reps

CHIN-UPS

Recommended Sets: 3 sets

Reps: 12 15 reps

BARBELL SHOULDER PRESS

Recommended Sets: 3 sets

Reps: 10 12 reps

BICEPS CURLS

Recommended Sets: 3 sets

Reps: 10 15 reps

SIDE DELT RAISES

Recommended Sets: 3 sets

Reps: 15 20 reps

WARMDOWN

Stretching 2 to 5 minutes

Day 2: Resistance Training for Lower Body

WARM-UP

Skipping /jogging for 3-6 minutes

SQUAT

Recommended Set: 3 sets

Reps: 8 10 reps

LEG EXTENSIONS

Recommended Set: 3 sets

Reps: 10 15 reps

LEG CURLS

Recommended Set: 3 sets

Reps: 10 15 reps

DEADLIFT

Recommended Set: 3 sets

Reps: 8 10 reps

STANDING CALF RAISES

Recommended Set: 3 sets

Reps: 15 reps

AB ROLLER

Recommended Set: 3 sets

Reps: -

WARMDOWN

Slow walk for about 2 -5 minutes

Day 3: REST

Day 4 Circuit Training for Upper Body

WARM-UP

Brisk-walk 3 5 minutes

DB SHOULDER PRESS

Recommended Reps: 10 12 reps

SEATED BICEPS CURLS

Recommended Reps: 10 15 reps

LAT PULLDOWN

Recommended Reps: 12 15 reps

TRICEPS PUSHDOWN

Recommended Reps: 15 20 reps

DUMBELL INCLINE BENCH PRESS

Recommended Reps: 8 10 reps

DUMBELL ONE ARM ROWS

Recommended Reps: 8 10 reps

REAR DELT RAISES

Recommended Reps: 15 20 reps

WARMDOWN

Slow walk for about 2 -5 minutes

NOTE: All exercises should be done in succession with 5 to 10 seconds rest intervals. Circuits should be done three times with 1 - 1½ minutes of rest, which may be difficult to achieve in a gym. Therefore, it is advisable to get the equipment handy or visit a specific group class in the gym to allow you to perform these exercises as advised.

Day 5: Circuit Training For Lower Body

WARM-UP

Skipping 2 minutes

GOBLET SQUAT

Recommended Reps: 8 10 reps

BULGARIAN SPLIT SQUATS

Recommended Reps: 10 15 reps

SEATED CALF RAISE

Recommended Reps: 15 reps

DEADLIFT WITH DUMBELLS

Recommended Reps: 8 10 reps

LYING HAMSTRING CURL

Recommended Reps: 10 15 reps

PLANKS

Recommended Reps: 30 seconds

WARMDOWN

Slow walk for about 2 -5 minutes

NOTE: All exercises should be done in succession with 5 to 10 seconds rest intervals. Circuits should be done three times with 1 - 1½ minutes of rest, which may be difficult to achieve in a gym. Therefore, it is advisable to get the equipment handy or visit a specific group class in the gym to allow you to perform these exercises as advised.

Day 6:

WARM-UP

Skipping /jogging for 3-6 minutes

30 minutes low-intensity steady-state cardio [LISS Cardio]

WARMDOWN

Day 7: REST

In summary, it is common knowledge that endomorphs gain weight easily but have difficulty losing fat due to their high-fat levels and slow metabolic rate. Other than cutting down calories, another way to burn calories, build muscle mass, and increase metabolism is by engaging in regular resistance training and exercise. Exercises such as plyometric box jumps, HIIT, running sprints, and skipping are some of the recommended exercises that can help you lose fat and build muscle.

To ensure that you do not regain lost weight, you should engage in other low-intensity exercises such as walking. In conclusion, you must burn about 300 calories per day more than you eat and exercise for about thirty to forty-five minutes daily.

Mesomorph

Mesomorphs can be regarded as the least problematic body type. This is because, unlike the other body types, they seem to have things in place efficient metabolic rate, fit body, well-built muscles, etc. And as a result of this, they require minimal to no effort in achieving their fitness goals. A study revealed that mesomorphs are fast in responding to stimuli, hence with little exercise, they can get a spike of about sixty percent in their muscle growth.

Although people may get this body type due to genetic factors, there are some essential steps to put into place to ensure the maintenance of this body. These steps include a healthy diet and exercise.

As a mesomorph, your protein intake should depend on the intensity of the exercise plan you have chosen. However, your regular protein intake should be between one and two grams per kilogram or 2 lbs of body weight regardless of this. You can get the remaining required calories for the body's daily function from a healthy diet that consists of fats and carbs.

Exercise Tips

Here are some tips to help you effectively go through your exercise program.

➢ **Exercise Frequency**: Relying on how easily mesomorphs can stimulate their muscle mass, it is recommended that they engage in exercises between three to four times weekly.

➢ **Exercise Reps**: A moderate range of reps is recommended to avoid injuries resulting from over-exercising.

A high probability that mesomorphs would need to introduce a supplement to their exercise plans. This is because relying on cardio exercises alone may not be sufficient to reach the desired goal.

Sample Exercise Plan

This section consists of a 7-days exercise plan for a mesomorph. It covers a sample exercise plan for both weight loss and building muscle.

Exercise Plan For Weight Loss

These exercises are cardiovascular exercises that are recommended for weight loss. However, for an effective result, it can be combined with weight training.

Day 1:

WARM-UP

SKIPPING 2 minutes

SCISSORS KICK

Recommended Set: 3 sets

Reps: 12 reps

CROSSBODY MOUNTAIN CLIMBERS

Recommended Set: 2 sets

Reps: 25 reps

WARMDOWN

Day 2:

WARM-UP

Lunges - 15

CRUNCHES

Recommended Set: 2 sets

Reps: 12 reps

BURPEES

Recommended Set: 3 sets

Reps: 8 reps

WARMDOWN

Day 3: REST

Day 4:

WARM-UP

Skipping 2 minutes

SQUAT

Recommended Set: 3 sets

Reps: 8 10 reps

PLANKS

Recommended Set: 3

Reps: -

WARMDOWN

Day 5:

WARM-UP

Jogging 3 minutes

GOBLET SQUAT

Recommended Set: 3

Reps: 10 - 12

SIT-UP

Recommended Set: 2

Reps: 12 reps

WARMDOWN

Day 6:

WARM-UP

Walking-lunges 20

CYCLING 30 45 minutes

WARMDOWN

Day 7: REST

Exercise Plan For Building Muscle

These exercises are a combination of compound and heavy resistance training with varying rep ranges which will enhance muscle stimulation.

Day 1: Exercise for the Upper Body

WARM-UP

Torso twist 20 [10 for each side]

BENCH PRESS

Recommended Set: 3 sets

Reps: 4 6 reps

CHIN-UP

Recommended Set: 3 sets

Reps: 12 15 reps

BARBELL SHOULDER PRESS

Recommended Set: 3 sets

Reps: 8 10 reps

BARBELL BICEPS CURLS

Recommended Set: 3 sets

Reps: 6 8 reps

SKULL CRUSHERS

Recommended Set: 2 sets

Reps: 10 12 reps

DUMBELL ROWS

Recommended Set: 3 sets

Reps: 8 10 reps

SIDE DELT RAISES

Recommended Set: 3 sets

Reps: 15 20 reps

WARMDOWN

Day 2: Exercise for the Lower Body

WARM-UP
Shoulder rotation 15 [Forward and in reverse]

SQUAT
Recommended Set: 3 sets
Reps: 4 6 reps

AB ROLLERS
Recommended Set: 3 sets
Reps: -

LEG CURLS
Recommended Set: 3 sets
Reps: 10 -15 reps

DEADLIFT
Recommended Set: 3 sets
Reps: 8 10 reps

LEG EXTENSION
Recommended Set: 3 sets
Reps: 10 15 reps

STANDING CALF RAISES
Recommended Set: 3 sets

Reps: 15 reps

WARMDOWN

Day 3 : REST

Day 4: Exercise for the Upper Body

WARM-UP

Walking lunges - 15

DUMBELL SHOULDER PRESS

Recommended Reps: 6 8 reps

SEATED BICEPS CURLS

Recommended Reps: 10 15 reps

LAT PULLDOWN

Recommended Reps: 12 15 reps

TRICEPS PUSHDOWN

Recommended Reps: 15 20 reps

DUMBELL INCLINE BENCH PRESS

Recommended Reps: 8 10 reps

REAR DELT RAISES

Recommended Reps: 15 20 reps

WARMDOWN

Day 5: Exercise for the lower body [2]

WARM-UP

Skipping 2 minutes

FRONT SQUAT

Recommended Reps: 8 10 reps

SEATED CALF RAISE

Recommended Reps: 15 reps

BULGARIAN SPLIT SQUATS

Recommended Reps: 10 12 reps

LYING HAMSTRING CURL

Recommended Reps: 10 12 reps

BARBELL DEADLIFT

Recommended Reps: 4 6 reps

PLANKS

Recommended Reps: 30 seconds

Day 6: REST

Day 7: REST

Since male mesomorphs are prone to easily gaining weight, a mixture of cardio and weight training is highly recommended. This is because their exercise focus should be on reducing their percentage of body fat. On the other hand, female mesomorphs should incorporate weight training into their daily routine since their primary goal is maintaining their body shape and toning.

In summary, cardio is essential in regulating fat levels. Hence, engaging in regular cardiovascular exercises is an effective means to avoid gaining excess weight. Therefore, thirty minutes of cardio two to three times weekly is recommended for mesomorphs.

Ectomorph

The lean frame and highly active metabolic body that ectomorphs have, make it difficult to gain or maintain weight. Therefore, their exercise routine should primarily consist of hypertrophy and maximal strength resistance exercises. However, unlike fast-paced aerobic activities that stimulate elevated calorie burn, strength resistance exercises and hypertrophy are anaerobic. Therefore, they won't enable elevated calorie burn, especially when combined with long periods of rest. Also, it is advised to adopt a diet with balanced fats, carbs, and high protein for optimal muscle growth.

Also, cardio training should be limited. Ectomorphs are prone to burn calories quickly; hence, to prevent muscle loss, cardiorespiratory exercises should be done carefully and within limits (30 minutes LISS or HIIT three times a week).

Exercise Tips

Here are some tips to help you effectively go through your exercise program.

➤ **Exercise Frequency**: Exercises are important in 'sculpting' your desired body shape. Therefore, as an ectomorph, it is recommended that you workout or engage in exercises at least four times a week. However, to get the most from these sessions, it is essential to focus on medium to high volume exercises by engaging in 3 to 5 sets and 8 to 12 reps of each exercise. You should also note that your workout should be between 30 minutes to 1 hour [including warm-up and warm-down].

➤ **Exercise Tools**: Unlike the other body types, ectomorphs need to add more load to their workouts to achieve similar results compared to the other body types. Therefore, it is recommended that they train with heavy weights to encourage muscle growth.

➤ **Exercise Routine**: When exercising as an ectomorph for weight or muscle gain, you will have to consider an exercise plan that is more about helping you achieve your desired body and not just an exercise that you are comfortable with.

➤ **Compound Movements**: In working towards achieving your body goals, it is important to focus on compound movements rather than isolated movements. The goal should be to engage multiple muscle groups to ensure maximum load and efficiency during your workouts. Some examples of these movements are bench-pressing, deadlifts, and squats.

Sample Exercise Plan

This section consists of a 7-days exercise plan for ectomorphs. These exercises combine compound movements and resistance training, which will help build a desirable body. In making a workout plan, it is advisable to include high-volume compound lifts.

Day 1: Exercise For Chest And Triceps

WARM-UP

Lunges 15

INCLINED DUMBELL PRESS

Recommended Set: 4 sets

Reps: 8 12 reps

DIPS

Recommended Set: 3 sets

Reps: 12 reps

OVERHEAD EXTENSIONS

Recommended Set: 4 sets

Reps: 8 12 reps

DUMBBELL FLYERS FLAT BENCH

Recommended Set: 3 sets

Reps: 12 reps

WARM DOWN

Day 2: Exercise For Back And Biceps

WARM-UP

Brisk walk 2 -5 minutes

SEATED BARBELL CURLS

Recommended Set: 4 sets

Reps: 8 10 reps

WIDE-GRIP PULL-UP

Recommended Set: 4 sets

Reps: 8 12 reps

BENT-OVER DUMBBELL ROWS

Recommended Set: 4 sets

Reps: 8 12 reps

ALTERNATE DUMBELL CURLS

Recommended Set: 3 sets

Reps: 12 reps

WARMDOWN

Day 3: Exercise For Legs And Shoulders

WARM-UP

Torso twist [10 for each side]

DEADLIFTS

Recommended Set: 3 sets

Reps: 12 reps

LATERAL RAISE

Recommended Set: 3 sets

Reps: 12 reps

BARBELL SQUATS

Recommended Set: 3 sets

Reps: 12 reps

LEG PRESS

Recommended Set: 4 sets

Reps: 8 12 reps

MILITARY PRESS

Recommended Set: 4 sets

Reps: 8 12 reps

LYING LEG CURLS

Recommended Set: 4 sets

Reps: 8 -12 reps

WARMDOWN

Day 4: Rest

Day 5: Total Body Superset

WARM-UP

Jogging 3 minutes

SKULL CRUSHERS

Recommended Set: 3 sets

Reps: 12 reps

PUSH-UP

Recommended Set: 3 sets

Reps: 12 reps

STANDING BICEP CURLS

Recommended Set: 3 sets

Reps: 12 reps

LAT PULLDOWN

Recommended Set: 3 sets

Reps: 12 reps

SHOULDER PRESS

Recommended Set: 3

Reps: 12

WARMDOWN

Day 6: Rest

Day 7: Rest

In conclusion, body type is a component that is often neglected in modern exercise plans, and this is because there are so many options available on the internet. People lose sight of the reality that their bodies are unique. Indeed, there is no 'one-size-fits-all' exercise plan for any of the different body types out there. Therefore, it is essential to recognize that you have a unique body type that influences your metabolism and your fitness goals in the long run.

The focus of endomorphs shouldn't just be on losing weight but also on boosting metabolism, which will prevent calories from being converted to fat. Since cardiovascular exercise keeps the body from returning to fat-storing mode, it is recommended as the most beneficial exercise for ectomorphs. Also, ectomorphs should include high-intensity interval training (HIIT) activities in their exercise routine. This is because HIIT has been proven to be an excellent way to stimulate fat burning that lasts long after exercise sessions.

While an ectomorph may prefer endurance activities like running, it is advisable to include resistance training. For example, including bodyweight or weight training may reduce your risk of injury while also helping you build muscles. Maintaining a healthy weight also requires high-intensity interval training. It helps stimulate both your aerobic and anaerobic cardio systems while improving your strength and muscle growth. An ectomorph diet must be well-balanced to help build strong muscles.

There is a popular view that mesomorphs do not have to exercise due to their natural muscular bodies. This is only a myth, and as a mesomorph, it is recommended that you exercise regularly [cardio or weightlifting] to maintain your physique. Mesomorphs have a natural propensity to develop muscle, and sports that require strength are reasonably easy for them to learn. Also, it is recommended that mesomorphs change their exercise routine or intensity from time to time [every 2 to 3 months] to stay in shape and also avoid a fitness plateau.

In addition, you should note that the whole point isn't just about engaging in exercises as you would do a chore. It is more about staying active. You can keep things interesting and challenging by including yoga, taking long walks outdoors, and playing an outdoor or indoor sport. What's critical here is to incorporate exercise (in whatever form) into your daily lives to ensure it becomes a healthy and positive habit that will have lasting effects on your health and wellbeing.

CHAPTER 5:
INTERMITTENT FASTING

There is another means of losing weight that complements the traditional methods [exercising and dieting]. It is known as intermittent fasting [IF]. Although this may likely surprise you at first, numerous nutritionists and dietitians swear by its effectiveness in losing weight in a healthy way.

Intermittent fasting has become is a popular health and weight-loss strategies. It involves alternating between regular fasting and periods of little to no food consumption. It primarily involves food restriction and food timing. The concept of IF is more concerned with when you should eat rather than what you eat. Therefore, it cannot be described as a diet but an eating strategy.

The two key components that make up IF are the length of the fast and the window of opportunity to consume the required calories. During the eating phase, which immediately follows the fasting period, you can consume the required daily calories of your meal plan while adhering to the fasting rules.

Please bear in mind that IF is not a miracle weight-loss method. Therefore, you shouldn't expect to lose all the excess fat you've gained as soon as you start to follow the eating plan. However, persevering with IF in conjunction with your diet and exercise plan will help you achieve your desired results.

There are many available nutritional methods of IF ranging from a few hours to days, and after consulting with your medical practitioner, you should choose the most beneficial one. For example, if you are a busy person with little or no time to have a healthy meal or engage in workouts, IF may be a viable alternative for you to explore. If, on the other hand, you are a food lover who is always conscious of the food in your surroundings, adopting other healthy eating habits that are more focused on the kind of nutrients that you consume will be more helpful for you.

When it comes to your quest for better health, IF should be a component of your entire strategy. It is normal if the question "why should I fast?" has crossed your mind when you contemplate the agony you must endure while fasting, especially if you are a beginner. However, an easy way to let go of that thought is to look on the brighter side of the many benefits you would derive from IF. Some of the benefits include the power to control your hunger, increased metabolism, optimal maintenance level of glucose level in the blood, reduced blood pressure, etc.

With intermittent fasting, you do not need to worry about purchasing a particular kind of food with a number of calories. Therefore, when you choose to be aware of your eating habits, your fasting strategy is more achievable, and you will maintain the desired results.

Therefore before you begin IF, you must understand the foundations upon which it is built, how it works, the different methods, the pros, and the cons. However, you must maintain an unwavering commitment to achieving your goal regardless of how difficult the journey may be. Focus on providing the best possible care for your body, have a committed mindset, and incorporate regular exercise into your lifestyle.

History Of Intermittent Fasting

Like every other concept, to fully understand the concept of Intermittent Fasting (IF), it is essential to understand its origin and how it evolved into what it is today. Therefore, this section aims to cover the evolution of IF.

Fasting has been used for religious purposes, extending lifespan, improving health, and many other purposes through the ages. It has been referenced in the sacred texts of many of the world's most prominent religions and by famous philosophers and great thinkers who all believe that fasting is beneficial to the point that they advocated that it be used as a method for healing the sick.

There is a popular misconception that fasting is all about self-deprivation, starvation, and hunger, which is untrue. Instead, fasting is a deliberate act to restrict food intake for a specified period. One chooses to undertake a strategy for many reasons, including health, religion, and others.

Fasting developed from different regions around the world, and the reasons for fasting vary from one location or person to another. Consequently, people don't only fast to lose weight. Fasting has been adopted for other reasons, such as improving concentration, avoiding Alzheimer's disease, delaying the aging process, and preventing insulin resistance. In addition, some individuals fast for religious reasons or as part of cultural traditions.

Numerous philosophers promoted the idea of fasting. One of them was Plutarch, a Greek writer, and an ancient historian. He expressed his belief in the power of fasting when he wrote, "Instead of using medicine, better fast today" in one of his books. Other philosophers that shared his belief were Philip Paracelsus, famous for his words, "the best of all medicines is resting and fasting," Aristotle, Plato, and Hippocrates of Cos.

In ancient Greece, nature was generally regarded as a source of healing. When we are ill, it is natural for our bodies to reject or have little interest in food. Fasting is thus viewed as a form of internal healing. When we consider our current environment, we realize that the last thing on our minds is food or eating when we are ill. As a result, fasting may be seen as a predisposition for almost every illness. However, fasting can be considered a normal tendency in the vast majority of health situations. Thus, they were numerous beliefs about fasting among the ancient Greeks.

Fasting is respected in many religions, including Christianity, Islam, Buddhism, and others. It is seen as a method that is inherently helpful to the human body in terms of eliminating toxins and increasing alertness and the mind to foster awareness and strengthen the mind-body connection.

Religious individuals fast in a variety of ways. For example, every day, Buddhists fast from noon till the dawn of the next day. The majority of the time, they eat in the morning and then fast for approximately 18 hours. They also go on water fasts for a few days or weeks at a time. Christians have no specific fasting routine, although some engage in a fast during 'Lent.'

The holy month of Ramadan is a month of fasting for Muslims. It entails going without meals from daybreak until dusk. This differs from other types of fasting in which fluid intake is restricted or completely prohibited. However, the phase where they are likely to experience moderate dehydration is common among the different fasting methods.

Fasting has been practiced for thousands of years and has withstood the test of time. A trial was recently carried out to put this history to the test in confirming the effectiveness of fasting in relation to weight.

The study was carried out on mice by Satchidananda Panda in 2012. The conclusion was that mice fed a high-fat diet for eight hours a day were much healthier and slimmer than mice who ate whenever they pleased. However, even though both groups consumed the same calories, the results were not the same. The study also indicated that time had an impact on the outcomes, leading to the coining of the phrase Time-Restricted Feeding (TRF).

After the successful research on the mice, Satchidananda Panda decided to replicate the study on humans to see if the results were the same. The human study was carried out in a variety of situations designed to simulate the real world. They used an obese group of men and women who had tried various diets high in sugar and fat. They observed that TRF was beneficial since it prevented health issues such as inflammation, high cholesterol, and insulin resistance regardless of the meals they consumed. The results from this study revealed that although fasting has been around for a long time, it was still beneficial. Hence, it is safe to say this concept is tested and trusted.

Intermittent Fasting Methods

Intermittent Fasting (IF) methods refer to the different ways in which an individual executes their fast. There are different fasting methods that every individual can adopt to suit themselves and their health needs. A common feature of all these other methods is splitting the fasting phase into two phases   The fasting phase   where there is a limiting of caloric intake, and the eating phase   where there is a controlled caloric intake. The acceptable pattern is to make your eating phase between 6 am and 6 pm while you fix your fasting period between 6 pm and 6 am.

The 16/8 Method

If an individual has their last meal at 8 pm and does not eat until noon the following day, technically, they have completed a 16/8 fast.

The 16/8 method is also known as the Lean gain method. This method is a common fasting method as most of the fast is completed while you are asleep. Also, many people tend to skip breakfast due to their busy schedules or for other reasons. The 16/8 method involves a fasting period of about 16 hours and limits your food consumption phase to 8 hours daily. During this food consumption phase, you can eat your desired calories in line with your fitness goals, which can be broken down into multiple meals. The easiest way to implement the 16/8 fasting method is to skip breakfast and avoid eating anything after 8 pm.

Unlike other fasting methods, the 16/8 approach is flexible as it relies on a time-restricted feeding pattern. The time frame opportunity phase is a personal choice. For example, you can choose to skip breakfast or choose to eat breakfast and then fast for 16 hours if you know you're going to be awake during the night. Research revealed that combining a TRF pattern such as the 16/8 method and resistance training helps to reduce fat and prevent hypertension.

However, this fasting method may not be easy for those who have major hunger cravings in the morning and find it extremely difficult to skip breakfast. During your opportunity phase, it is critical to eat mostly balanced and nutritious meals comprising vegetables, proteins, fruits, healthy fats, and whole grains to enhance the health benefits of this eating pattern. If you eat a lot of unhealthy snacks, junk foods, or processed foods, this method may likely not experience a positive effect of this method. On the other hand, you can consume coffee, other low-calorie liquids, and water to help you feel less hungry during the fast. It is best to set a caloric intake limit and eat in accordance with this limit.

A high-protein diet is ideal for an individual adopting the 16/8 method as it helps retain lean muscle. However, there must be a relative increase in the number of carbs in your diet on the days you intend to exercise compared to the days when you rest. Therefore, your first meal must contain a significant percentage of your total calories for that day following your workout. Following this fast method for a week means that you will fast for about 112 hours every week, which will help you lose fat fast provided you are eating within your caloric limit and eating healthy whole foods.

Eat-Stop-Eat Method

This method involves fasting for a precise 24 hour period. For example, eating breakfast at 8 am on day one and not eating anything else till 8 am on day two.

This method is also known as One day fast. This means that you can pick a relaxing day of the week to stay away from food altogether. For example, you can decide to abstain from food from breakfast, lunch, or dinner one day until breakfast, lunch, or dinner the next day. Although no solid food is permitted during the fast, low-calorie liquids, coffee, and water are allowed.

However, for the remaining six days, you can continue with your usual eating pattern. Although there is a tendency that one may want to fill up on the calories they lost or will lose during the fast, it is recommended that you avoid overconsumption and stick to a balanced diet.

The concept of this method is to help you lose weight by reducing your total weekly calories consumption. For example, if an individual has a total weekly calorie intake of about 8500 calories, that would drop to 7300 (1200 lower) the week they perform a 24 hour or eat-stop-eat fast.

Research has proven that the 24 hours fast can lead to a metabolic shift that is capable of causing the body to burn fat for energy rather than carbs [glucose]. However, as beneficial as this appears, this fasting method requires strong willpower. Therefore, it is vital to seek medical advice before adopting this fasting method.

The Warrior Diet Method

This method of fasting was one of the first popular diets that included a form of intermittent fasting. It is based on the eating habits of ancient warriors, also known as 20/4. This means that the fasting period is 20 hours and the eating period is 4 hours. It primarily involves fasting for most of the day and then consuming your required calories during the eating period. You should also note that there is no specific eating period. Therefore you can choose your 4-hours eating window at any time during the day or night.

In intermittent fasting, the warrior diet method of fasting appears to be the best for beginners. This is because it is easy to go from your regular eating pattern to the warrior diet. You may start by taking fewer calories during the fasting period before having a proper meal during the eating period. This is an excellent choice for those who like large meals with high-calorie content.

The Warrior Diet recommends eating small amounts of dairy products, hard-boiled eggs, and non-calorie beverages during the fasting period. When you break your fast, your first snacks should be vegetables, water, and healthy fruits. Also, to ensure that you maintain consistent caloric intake, your main meal should contain unprocessed foods, healthy fats, and a lot of protein.

This method of fasting is more severe than the 16/8 method but less strict than the Eat-Stop-Eat approach. Although it may be challenging to begin with this fasting method, you must make every effort to avoid eating any meals outside of the eating period. For example, instead of fasting one day and then eating breakfast and lunch the next, it is recommended to be consistent with your eating pattern.

The 5/2 Diet Method

This fasting method is straightforward. It involves following your regular eating pattern five days a week. Then you limit your calories to about one-quarter of your usual daily caloric intake for the remaining two days. This is usually around 500 calories for women and 600 for men.

A possible scenario to implement this diet would be to fast on a Monday and Thursday. You would eat three small meals that day to make up your 'lowered' calories and eat normally the remaining five days.

You should note that this fasting method doesn't specify the days of the week in which you can decide to limit your calories. Also, there is no restriction on when or what to eat during your eating period. Although, it is recommended that you eat healthily. Eat healthy whole foods to ensure that the lower calories are used wisely to keep yourself from feeling hungry too soon.

Several studies have proven that this fasting method plays a vital role in assisting with weight reduction. It has also been proven to be as efficient as a continuous calorie restriction diet in preventing metabolic diseases such as diabetes and heart diseases.

Although the 5/2 fasting method may be beneficial, it is important to consult a doctor before adopting this method.

Alternate Day Fast Method

This fasting method involves fasting every other day. It simply involves eating what you want one day and fasting the next. You can consume low/no-calorie drinks in abundance on diet days, including water, black coffee, and tea.

This method will involve going to bed on an empty stomach on fasting days at least three times a week. Hence, it is not advisable for beginners as it may seem rather extreme.

There are different versions of the alternate-day fast, each version with its specification. While some versions suggest that there should be a total restriction of calories, some other versions suggest that you should limit the calories consumed during the fasting period to about 500 calories, which is an excellent way to ease yourself into this diet.

Fasting on alternate days has been proven to help in weight reduction. According to recent research, the combination of alternate-day fasting and endurance exercise may result in weight reduction that is twice as effective as fasting alone. In addition, a study on obese individuals revealed that alternate-day fasting was equally as efficient at decreasing body weight as daily calorie restriction.

Whether you start with a modified fasting schedule or a complete fast, eating a balanced diet that includes vegetables low in calories and high-protein meals is important to prevent you from always getting hungry.

Skipping Meals

There are other methods of Intermittent Fasting that don't necessarily include strict schedules. This primarily involves skipping meals spontaneously. Alternatively, you may skip meals occasionally, such as when you are too busy to make a meal or when you aren't very hungry.

You are following a spontaneous intermittent fast when you skip one or two meals on the spur of the moment. So, if you don't feel like eating breakfast one day, skip it and replace it with a nutritious lunch or dinner. The key is that you are eating well-balanced and healthy meals during your eating period.

In conclusion, every technique has the potential to be helpful, but determining which one is best for you is a question of individual preference, lifestyle, and experience. The goal is always to lose excess body fat and reach a healthy body weight.

Although these techniques would help you lose weight by lowering your calorie consumption, you mustn't compensate by eating excess calories during the eating period. Fasting for the first time may be challenging, so start slowly and gradually extend the duration of your fasting period as your endurance improves. To get the desired effects, you must arrange a fast that fits your daily routine and lifestyle.

As with any fasting technique, practice awareness and completely engage yourself in your daily activities.

Stages Of Fasting

During intermittent fasting, your body experiences several changes depending on the rate at which you fast. Some of these changes are physical - evident weight loss, while others are internal - improved glucose control. During your fasting phase, your body goes through a cycle primarily characterized by changes in hormonal levels and metabolism. The stages include the fed state, early fasting state, fasting state, and long-term fasting state. The variance in all these fasting stages is found in how they affect hormonal levels, their primary source of energy, and their metabolic rate.

The Fed State

This refers to the first few hours after you eat a meal, leaving your body to digest and absorb the nutritional components of the meal.

During the fed state, there is an increase in the amount of insulin secreted. Insulin is the hormone that transports sugar from the bloodstream into the cells. The amount of insulin released is based on your body's sensitivity to insulin and the nutritional components of the meal consumed. Also, there is an increase in the blood sugar level where stored carbs can be converted back to sugar when the body needs it for fuel.

Other hormones such as Leptin [the hormone responsible for suppressing appetite] increase during this state while Ghrelin, [the hormone which stimulates hunger] decreases when you eat.

In conclusion, the nutritional composition of your meal and the portion of the meal consumed determines how long your body stays in the fed state.

Early Fasting State

The early fasting state starts around 3-4 hours after a meal and lasts about 18 hours. Common fasting methods such as the 16/8 method of fasting fall between the fed and the early fasting state.

In this state, the body converts amino acids into energy. Also, the body converts glycogen (energy reserve for glucose) into sugar to use as energy as the insulin level, and blood sugar levels decline. The body slowly runs out of glycogen towards the end of this state and begins to find an alternative energy source.

Fasting State

This state runs from 18 hours to 48 hours of fasting, depending on your preferred fasting method.

During this state, the body begins to break down stored up protein and fats as its alternative source of energy. This process causes the body to transit into a metabolic state known as Ketosis.

However, certain factors that may include genetics, the composition of your meal, and your food portion may affect the rate at which your body enters into Ketosis. This means that you shouldn't expect to enter Ketosis immediately after your body transits into the fasting state. Also, you should note that unless you include very low carbs meals in your diet, fasting methods with fasting periods of less than 18 hours is not sufficient to push the body into Ketosis.

Long-Term Fasting State

This state usually occurs in an extended period of fasting. It starts around 48 hours after your last meal. There is a steady rise in the level of beta-hydroxybutyrate [BHB] during this state, while there is a continuous decrease in insulin level.

BHB is a chemical produced by the body to supply energy when its primary source of energy (sugar or carbs) is low. Also, there is a reduction in the breaking down of protein to help protect the muscle tissues in the body. The primary source of energy in this state is sugar generated from the kidney.

Fasting Rules

There are certain fundamental rules designed to guide beginners on intermittent fasting. Therefore, it is important to follow these rules to avoid the common mistakes associated with IF.

When To Eat

As you already know, IF is all about timing your meal. Hence, the first step is to choose a fasting method. This will help you determine how long your fasting period will last. However, as a beginner, it is not advisable to choose methods with long fasting periods.

The next step after choosing a fasting method is to select a time frame. This means you can pick a comfortable time frame that would serve as the fasting and eating periods. Also, it is essential to stick to the fasting rules by avoiding food when you are in your fasting period.

What To Eat

Although calorie deficit significantly impacts weight loss, Intermittent Fasting is a flexible eating pattern that doesn't require a specific diet.

The common reason Intermittent Fasting is recommended is to help you lose weight by re-arranging your caloric consumption. Therefore, it is highly recommended that you consume whole foods that will keep you full for longer and put your body in the best state to benefit from the effects of fasting. Junk food usually has higher calories and lower nutritional value, which will be counter-productive to the effects of IF. It may help to seek advice from a qualified nutritionist to help you optimize your meals that best suit your fasting strategy.

When To Exercise

Research has proven that the best time to exercise is during the fasting time frame, as the body is more likely to utilize the body's stored fat reserves for fuel. However, it is important to exercise in a controlled manner to avoid exhaustion during workouts.

Pros And Cons

Intermittent Fasting (IF) is an excellent technique for reducing body weight since it has many advantages for both your body and your mind. In addition, how you choose to fast may have negative consequences on your health.

> ➤ **WEIGHT LOSS**: Although there is no rule enforcing counting calories in IF, the concept is largely based on cutting calories. Since all the different fasting methods incorporate skipping meals and eating fewer calories, it will prove difficult for most individuals to consume all the required calories

within their eating period. Hence, it is inevitable that you will lose belly fat and body weight in the long run.

In 2014, research was conducted on humans to know the impact of IF on weight loss. The result revealed about a 3% 8% reduction in body weight within a period of three to twenty-four weeks. The research also revealed that the rate at which a person on IF lost weight weekly was approximately 0.25 0.75 kg/ 0.55   1.65   lbs.   In addition, there was an indication that they lost belly fat. However, it is important to mention that these results will only be possible if you avoid overeating and compensating for calories lost while you are on the fast.

> **Easy Eating Plan**: A survey on IF revealed that many people adopted it as their weight loss strategy because of its simplicity. Other than timing your meal, IF does not have strict requirements like other weight loss plans. It makes eating healthily, more manageable, and straightforward.

> **Cellular Repair**: As soon as your body enters the fasting state, the cells in your body initiate a repair process. Autophagy is a good illustration of this. This process refers to a cell's ability to break down proteins while simultaneously removing old ones accumulated inside the cell.

> **Heart Health**: IF is beneficial for metabolic health. It also plays a role in reducing the risk of cardiovascular disease by reducing the risk factors

blood sugar, cholesterol, inflammatory markers, and insulin resistance.

> **Brain Health**: IF helps to prevent Alzheimer's disease. It may also aid in the development of new nerve cells.

IF results in low insulin levels, which allows the body to be more sensitive to even small incremental changes in insulin levels, which is beneficial.

However, in certain instances, IF may be harmful to your health and not suitable for everyone.

Research has shown that when you begin IF, you may feel fatigued, and your brain may not function as effectively as it used to. Hunger is the most reported side effect, but nausea and vomiting are also typical occurrences. However, this may be a temporary situation because your body will need to adapt to the new eating pattern.

According to some research, women may not benefit as much from intermittent fasting as men do. In addition, some women had claimed that their periods/menstrual cycle stopped when they started IF and returned to normal when they resumed their previous eating patterns.

Therefore, these are some of the reasons why women should approach intermittent fasting with caution. If they have any problems, such as menstrual irregularities, they should also stop immediately. In addition, avoid intermittent fasting if you are pregnant, breastfeeding, experiencing reproductive issues, or trying to conceive.

You should seek medical advice before starting an IF program. Especially if you are under medication, have an underlying medical condition such as diabetes or low blood pressure, have a history of eating disorders or blood sugar control issues, are underweight, or have a history of other health issues.

However, according to the American Heart Association, intermittent fasting has a very good safety record but should be implemented with caution.

Intermittent Fasting And You

IF as a beginner may appear challenging at first. This is why it is essential to understand the process before implementing it in your daily schedule. This section consists of tips that will help you achieve your fitness goals via IF.

> ➢ **Timing**: Intermittent Fasting is a program that requires research and understanding before one implements it. You can start your fasting journey once every two weeks and gradually progress once your body starts getting used to this change. You can also tailor your IF to best suit your lifestyle and how your body responds.

> ➢ **Calories**: As much as you are advised to eat normally during your eating period, you must avoid overeating. You shouldn't compensate or try to stock up on the calories you missed during your fasting period. Also, at the beginning of IF, counting calories is not a requirement; however, if

you experience a stall, you can incorporate calorie counting into your fasting plan.

➤ **Food Quality**: Although there is no recommended diet in IF, it is recommended that you maintain a healthy diet consisting of nutritious and whole foods and steer clear of junk or processed food. Give your body the best chance to succeed in the most timely and efficient way possible.

➤ **Exercise**: Inactivity can lead to excess weight gain. Therefore, it is vital to keep the body active. This can be done by including exercises such as strength training in your weight loss strategy. For people who are too busy to engage in exercises, you can include indoor (a swim during your lunch break) or outdoor activities (quick tennis game after work) in your daily schedule.

➤ **Consistency**: It is necessary to remain consistent with your fasting rules to achieve your goals.

➤ **Patience**: This cannot be overemphasized that IF is not a magic pill, so you can't expect to achieve your goals overnight. It takes strict adherence and commitment to the rules, consistency, and patience to achieve your desired body.

Also, it would help you if you kept in mind that people will always respond differently to a set of stimuli. As a result, before starting any IF program, you should first study your body and evaluate whether it is suitable for your body type.

For example, various studies have revealed that body types more sensitive to carbs like mesomorph and endomorphs are likely to enjoy the weight loss benefits attached to IF.

Ectomorphs struggle with gaining and maintaining body fat; therefore, fasting for prolonged periods is not recommended. Their structural composition already lacks fat, and fasting for an extended period will only cause them to lose more fat or muscle. However, since fasting provides other health benefits, they can fast for a short period to see how it works. For example, they can engage in 12 hours of fasting once or at most twice a week. It is also recommended that they get their calories during their eating period from nutrient-dense foods, especially proteins and carbs.

Mesomorphs are commonly referred to as the 'in-between' body type. However, you should note that mesomorphs can either be looking to lose or gain weight. Therefore, it is important to study your body needs before you engage in IF. The 16/8 fasting method is recommended for beginners looking to lose weight and mesomorphs who fast for health benefits.

On the other hand, endomorphs appear to be the body type with the most difficulty losing weight. Therefore, it is recommended that they engage in long hours of fasting, although this is subject to medical advice. Alternate day fasting or One meal a day [OMAD] are the common recommendations for endomorphs. This is because fasting for longer hours helps to limit fat storage while it stabilizes insulin levels.

In summary, once you've mastered the elements of fasting, you will find it easy to adapt. First, it helps to shape the traditional mindset that your body requires food whenever you're hungry. When you fast, you are letting your body unwind from the continuous strain associated with digestion. During this phase, your body redirects the energy it expends digesting food to other beneficial uses. These include reducing the number of antigens your immune system must deal with, repairing your gut wall, and exponentially increasing the productivity of your digestive glands by reducing the stress that is constantly put on them.

During your fast, your digestive system is put to rest while the blood purifies itself, the stomach cleanses itself, and your mind is free to focus on other important parts of life other than eating. Therefore, it is essential to drink fluids while fasting to enhance the efficiency of the cleansing process.

If you decide to try IF, remember that the quality of your meals is critical to your success. Consuming processed food at mealtimes will not help you lose weight or improve your health and will be counter-productive to your efforts.

Additionally, individuals who have an eating problem or are at risk of developing one should refrain from IF. It may also be a problem for those who have underlying medical conditions. Therefore, before you start fasting, check with a medical professional to ensure you don't have any pre-existing medical conditions.

In conclusion, you have the choice to discontinue fasting after you have attained your desired body weight or continue fasting. Also, to assist you in keeping track of your weight loss, it is recommended that you get a journal to record your total calorie intake, fasting periods, and weight over time.

It may also help to switch from IF to going back to a regular diet to ensure your body and brain break from the pattern. Keep the body and mind guessing to provide the best results.

A Practical IF Scenario

For those of you looking to implement IF, here is a scenario to start with involving the 16/8 method, which means you only have an 8-hour window to eat.

- ➢ Begin by deciding when you go to sleep (for argument sake let's say 10pm)
- ➢ Now count back 2 hours (8pm)
- ➢ 8pm is when you stop eating. You will consume all your meals between 12pm and 8pm.
- ➢ Preferably consume 4 meals during this time.
- ➢ To 'super-charge' IF effects, try this pattern 7 days a week.
- ➢ It is likely you may fail initially. If you do, don't worry. Try to get back to this pattern and make sure you slowly improve.

On average it takes 3 weeks for your body to get used to this pattern.

Side Effects & How To Manage Them

When beginning any diet involving fasting your body is bound to experience some side effects. The main side effects include fatigue, headaches, feeling on edge and of course hunger.

You can mitigate most of these effects by drinking a lot of water and consuming unsweetened beverages like black coffee and green tea.

Also learn to live and adapt to these new feelings. Like everything in life mindset plays a huge part in achieving success. It's good to look at the effects of fasting as a positive and train your mind to focus on the long-term benefits rather than the short-term effects.

We often confuse boredom with hunger which is why we find ourselves eating more when sitting aimlessly on the couch watching TV. When our body start to settle into a routine around fasting, it is your mind that's retraining itself around hunger cues. Your meals will be more efficient when your body is replenishing itself, recycling waste and take a well-earned break from constantly digesting food.

It's best to stay active when embarking on a fast. Best time to do this would be at the start of the week when you're at work for the next 5 days rather than over the weekend.

CHAPTER 6:
FITNESS GOALS

I t is common for people to start making plans towards the end of one year for the following year. These plans are usually referred to as 'Resolutions.' Resolutions are often personal plans that cover different aspects of life such as career, finances, health, marriage, physiology, family, education, etc.

For example, in December 2019, an individual makes a fitness resolution to lose 25lbs by December 2020. However, when they revisited their resolution at the proposed time, they realized that they could not meet this goal, leading to negative thinking regarding their weight, body, and health in general.

Quite a number of people have faced this at some point in their lives. However, while it may appear as though not meeting your goals is entirely your fault, it might interest you to know that sometimes, it isn't just about caring enough or working hard enough to achieve these goals.

There is a recurring reason we fail to achieve our goals, and research has shown that many people are still oblivious to this. For example, it's easy to say, 'I want to lose weight or 'I want to get fit and then include a random time frame, but have you ever thought to ask yourself if these resolutions were realistic enough or if you were going about it the right way?

This chapter will provide the tips you need to set realistic fitness goals and achieve them with ease. It will also help you note your mistakes, help you correct and turn them into positive habits.

Common Weight Loss Mistakes

Five weeks after an individual began their fitness journey, they decided to check their progress but realized they had only lost two pounds. Before that day, they followed the 16/8 fasting method and exercised four times a week, but it was apparent it wasn't working.

Sometimes, losing weight appears difficult because you can't seem to achieve your goals despite following all the rules. Therefore, it is understandable that the moment people realize that they are in the same position described earlier, they feel like giving up.

Many people have failed to realize that the reason they struggle with losing weight despite knowing their body type and adopting the method that fits is that they take steps without verifying its authenticity. These steps have greatly hindered health goals, but people are oblivious of how it affects their fitness goals.

These mistakes will be categorized and discussed under the three weight loss methods mentioned in this book for easy understanding.

Dieting

The many misconceptions attached to dieting have formed a notion that can be regarded as the primary cause of people's mistakes in matters concerning food and diet. Some of these mistakes are:

Calories:

The mistakes involving calories usually have an adverse effect on overall health. Weight loss can only be guaranteed when you expend more calories than the total calories you consume   also known as a 'caloric deficit.' Although this is common knowledge, many people still do not correctly apply it to their meals. The typical impact of this is that you will most likely consume unhealthy ingredients, unwanted calories, and you would have no idea of the number of calories you're consuming. On the other hand, many people are unaware that a caloric deficit varies from one person to another. For example, Female B, who cuts out 450 calories from her daily consumption of 2000 calories, will have different results to Female A, who cuts her daily calorie consumption of 1900 calories by 450 calories. Another common mistake associated with a caloric deficit is over-restriction. Since a caloric deficit is an essential requirement for weight loss, people eat far too little. This affects the body's metabolic rate, and you will begin to lose muscle mass instead of losing fat.

What to Do: Too many calories hinder weight loss, and at the same time, too few calories make you hungry and can reduce your metabolism and muscle mass. Therefore, to balance this, it is crucial to maintain a journal or a tracking app to help you track your meals and caloric consumption. Tracking will help you stay aware and make adjustments where necessary.

Also, set a meal plan to help you avoid over-restriction. This meal plan could either be daily, weekly, or monthly. Chapter 4 of this book provides a 7-days meal plan sample for each body type.

Fat Diet:

A lot of people deliberately opt for a low-fat diet. They believe that since they are trying to get rid of fat, their meals should consist of little to no fat. However, it has been proven that other than increasing hunger, low-fat foods are usually loaded with hidden sugars.

What to Do: Although excess fat can prevent weight loss, ensure that your diet consists of nutritious and well-balanced meals.

Crash Dieting:

This involves rushing through a diet plan. Although you may reach your goal, you would cause a lot of harm to your body, and also, you are bound to regain all the weight you lost and even more.

What To Do: Patiently follow the rules of your diet and allow it to work as it should. That way, you are likely to get rid of the weight in a controlled manner and for the long term.

Mindless Eating:

A lot of people are guilty of this. Mindless eating refers to eating for reasons other than being hungry. It will most likely hinder your weight loss plans because you will eat more than your body requires. This could be stress eating, eating while binge-watching a television series, eating because you are bored or sad, eating for fun, etc.

What To Do: Only eat when you are hungry. Train your body and mind to eat at designated times. Stay hydrated so your body doesn't confuse these cues for hunger.

Exercise

Keeping your body active is crucial in your weight loss journey. One of the best things you can do to lose weight and ensure overall good health is to include exercise in your daily schedule. Exercising is beneficial because it helps reduce the risk of chronic diseases such as diabetes and heart diseases other than enhancing your physical abilities. However, this may not be the case for those who make mistakes in their exercise. Some of these common mistakes are:

Resistance Training:

Incorporate resistance training into your exercise schedule. Not only does resistance training improve physical strength, but it also tops the list of the most effective exercise techniques for gaining muscle and increasing metabolic rate.

WHAT TO DO: Combine aerobic exercise with resistance training. Examples are lunges, push-ups, swimming, etc. Note that weight lifting doesn't necessarily mean lifting heavyweights.

Warmup And Warm Down:

People just walk right into the gym and jump right into their workout session, and when they are done, they just walk out. It has been medically proven that this is not only wrong but also dangerous.

What To Do: Start and end your sessions with a light exercise such as skipping, jogging, etc. Also, to make it effective, you can focus more on the part of the body you plan to train that day. E.g., jogging before a lower-body workout.

Incorrect Technique:

Incorrect technique when starting as a beginner or even as a seasoned athlete can affect your desired results and, at worst, cause serious injury.

What To Do: Employ the services of a personal trainer or coach or sign up at a gym or watch exercise videos online. Always begin with low or no weights and progress gradually.

Over Exercising:

The pressure to lose weight may overwhelm you to the point that the only place anyone can find you is at the gym. As much as it is important to exercise, you shouldn't overdo it. This is because over-exercising defeats the purpose of training. Other than that, it may lead to severe stress and injury.

What To Do: Take one or two days off in a week as a 'rest' day to help you recover. A study has shown that over-exercising is not sustainable; hence, to ensure that you have a sustainable goal, make an exercise plan with the help of a fitness trainer. You can also check out Chapter 5 for a 7-day exercise sample plan for your unique body type.

Intermittent Fasting

In this method of weight loss, beginners have the highest record of mistakes. This is primarily characterized by the challenges attached to adjusting to a new pattern of eating. Some of these mistakes include

Gradual Implementation:

Most individuals looking to lose weight or fat want to achieve their goal in the fastest way possible. IF is no different. When you come across the concept, it appears simple enough, and most individuals would apply a method that doesn't fit well with their lifestyle or personality. Some techniques require practice, and when these are not gradually implemented, it may lead to failure and disappointment.

What To Do: Start by periodically skipping meals and then gradually ease into the method that suits your body.

Compensating:

Restricting your eating phase to a specific time and still consuming the same calories as you were previously defeats the purpose of IF. For example, an individual adopts the 16/8 fasting method and then breaks down their eating phase into four stages, consuming about 450 calories during each meal. This means that they consume a total of 1800 calories daily. However, their maintenance calories were 1800 before fasting. Those who fall into this category will likely weigh the same or even more than before they started IF.

What To Do: Since IF is a plan that helps you lose weight by reducing the number of times or hours you eat, you should cut out about 20% of your total daily calorie consumption and divide the remaining 80% across the meals you eat during your eating phase. In addition, you should ensure that 80% consists of whole and nutritious food.

Over Eating:

This isn't limited to eating more than your body needs or requires; it also involves eating the wrong meals. In this case, wrong meals refer to processed food and all other unhealthy meals.

What To Do: Keep your eating phase clean by consuming only well-balanced and nutritional meals. In addition, the length of your eating phase should determine the number of meals you eat during your eating phase. For example, if your eating phase is 4 hours, you should not have more than two meals and a snack.

Exercise:

Tailor your exercise routine to ensure it fits in with your fast. This means exercising just before a meal to ensure that your body regains nutrients lost from the workout and doesn't feel fatigued. Not incorporating exercise in the right way can also lead to injuries and muscle loss, which is counter-productive to your weight loss efforts.

What To Do: As much as it is important to incorporate exercises into your fast, you mustn't overdo it. Plan your exercise just as you would your diet. Seek professional help where required but make sure your exercise routine is complementing your diet and fast routine.

Dehydration:

Many people treat IF like a regular fasting plan that prohibits liquids, leaving them dehydrated, low on energy, and leading to major health problems.

What To Do: IF isn't the same as a 'dry' fast or other fasting methods where liquids are not allowed. Therefore, you are permitted to drink low-calorie, un-sweetened liquids like water, green tea, or black coffee during your fast to keep you hydrated.

Consuming Wrong Food:

Individuals may consume food that they believe is a healthy, wholesome food that may contain high fat or carbs that may not help with their overall weight loss as per their body type.

What To Do: Carefully read labels of products before you purchase or consume them. Also, inquire about ingredients that make up a meal you are buying or when someone else has cooked a meal for you.

You may lose focus and get off track in your IF program. What is key is that you don't make it a habit. It is also recommended that you occasionally and deliberately include 'cheat meals/days' where you can enjoy all your favorite meals, drinks, and snacks. This will motivate you and help you from slipping off.

How to Incorporate Cheat Meals Effectively

Although it is highly recommended to include "cheat days" in a strict diet, many people have failed to incorporate them effectively. This is why many people haven't gotten any significant results despite being committed to a weight loss diet plan. This act has led to a significant setback in their fitness and weight loss journey. Sometimes, this act is often a result of ignorance or being misinformed. This section is to help curb this setback.

When you are on a diet, there are quite several things your body does, and one of them includes fighting back. During a diet, the body fights back in the following ways:

> ➤ **Muscle glycogen level**: This is usually used for energy during your diet; hence the body causes a gradual decrease. This affects workout sessions as it causes a decrement in your overall performance.

> ➤ **Energy expenditure** causes you to burn fewer calories, and you do not move as much as you usually would, thereby decreasing your energy expenditure. This is harmful as it may lead to fat loss plateaus.

> ➤ **Hormone levels**: There is a considerable increase in your appetite due to the decrease in leptin hormone levels.

Cheat meals provide our minds with the psychological fuel to carry on with a strict diet. Therefore, it is recommended that you incorporate them into your eating plan by setting aside one day to 're-fuel.'

For example:

Maintenance calories = 2500

These calories are based on an individual's BMR.

Caloric Deficit (required for fat loss) = 2000 (minus 500 calories).

Day 1 = 2000 calories
Day 2 = 2000 calories
Day 3 = 2000 calories
Day 4 = 1800 calories(less by 700)

Day 5 = 1800 calories (less by 700)

Day 6 = 1800 calories (less by 700)

Day 7 = 3100 calories (plus 1000)

Ideally, your cheat meal should be a high-carb, low-fat meal. This is because carbs are known to have added benefits such as:

> **Refilling muscle glycogen**: Carbs helps to counter the negative effect of fighting back that your body has on your workout sessions. It can enhance anabolic response in your sessions. Carbs also help to create more muscle fullness.

> **Boosting leptin level**: Since the body causes a decrease in leptin level, carbs are essential to counter it. It can also help increase energy expenditure and suppress appetite to facilitate weight loss.

You should always be mindful whenever you decide to begin a diet. Calories add up quickly, so try and trick the mind with meals that compliment your diet. For example, you should drink black coffee rather than coffee with milk - this cuts down on simple calories which start to add up.

In summary, if you are in a hurry to lose fat, the probability that you will make one or more of the above mistakes is high and slow down, or at worse, stop your weight loss journey. However, you should note that it is never too late to correct an unhealthy lifestyle and transform it into a healthy one.

With motivation, discipline, and consistency, you can achieve your goals.

Smart Goals

Now that you know why you haven't experienced significant weight loss, the next step is to review your goals and put a plan in place to help you achieve these goals. When drafting these goals, it is important to keep your body type, age, and fitness level in mind.

SMART is an acronym for a five-step method that aids and supports fitness goals. People who include these characteristics in their fitness goals have had a record of efficiently achieving their fitness and life goals in general.

The acronym SMART stands for:

➢ **Specific**: The first step in creating a fitness goal is to ensure that your goal is specific. This enhances the possibility of success. After all, how will you know if you have achieved your goals if they are vague? For example, you can't say you want to lose weight and then start exercising without clearly defining the goal. Instead, you can say, "I want to lose 10 lbs/5kg in 5 weeks or lose 2 inches off my waist." The latter is a specific goal that you can start to visualize and plan for.

➢ **Measurable**: For you to be able to monitor and track your progress, you must set measurable fitness goals. A measurable goal must be coupled with a time frame to achieve the goal. For example, you may have to consider your workout duration and number of reps while exercising. An example of a measurable goal is 'I want to exercise four times every week.' Setting a measurable goal keeps you motivated.

➢ **Achievable**: Considering your current health and fitness level, do you think it is possible to achieve your goals within the stipulated time frame you attached to your goals? One of the easiest ways to set yourself up for disappointment is by setting unrealistic fitness goals. For example, losing weight might be a pressing issue for you, but it's illogical to want to start your fitness plan by adopting a 20/4 method of Intermittent Fasting. Instead, start by skipping breakfast or lunch, and then gradually progress from there. The best way to set an achievable fitness goal is to note down your abilities and limitations and then model your goals around them.

➢ **Relevant**: Before you make fitness plans, you must consider the significance of that goal to you or your lifestyle. This will help you determine if it is a relevant goal or not. For example, if you struggle to wake up in the morning, there is no point in signing up for morning classes in the gym or planning to go out for a run or walk in the morning. Ensure the relevance of your plan is tailored to who you are and your lifestyle. You're more inclined to stay motivated if your plan complements your lifestyle. You should note that the relevancy of a goal to your fitness plan is your motivation to go through with it.

➢ **Time-Bound**: It is an important characteristic of your goals. Every goal must include a time frame in which it must be achieved. This takes away any uncertainty with planning and helps the mind focus on the goal. However, your time frame has to be reasonable. You shouldn't attach too much time to a goal as you may slack, and too little time may make it impossible to achieve.

Some of the benefits of setting SMART goals include

➢ **Accountability**: It helps you to take responsibility for your actions. When you feel like you are slacking, you can always go back to your plans and make the necessary corrections.

➢ **Motivation**: Setting SMART goals makes it easier for you to remain motivated and pushes you to achieve the goals as and when due.

➢ **Reasonability**: SMART goals give an avenue to set realistic and attainable goals, making it possible to reach your target in the long run.

➢ **Progress Tracking**: Since you can include a time frame in your fitness plans, it will help you make a periodical review of how far you've progressed and what is left.

Once you've made a SMART fitness goal, you can start working on it by signing up at a gym or begin setting up a home gym. Anything you invest in, be it material or mental, is relative to your requirements. You will get what you give in terms of effort.

Fitness Journal

It's not surprising that when you hear or see 'journal,' the first thing that comes to mind is a book for keeping track of your daily activities or a to-do list. Over time, this is the opinion that has been formed in our society. Although this is in no way wrong, it may interest you to know that 'journal' or 'journaling' has different connotations for health and fitness.

A survey revealed that for those looking for an effective way to stay on top of their fitness goals, make lifestyle changes, and make the best of their health, a fitness journal is essential. This is because a fitness journal helps you keep track of your meals, workout sessions, daily mood, and overall health progress.

Furthermore, the study conducted in the AMIA Annual Symposium Proceedings revealed that keeping a log routine of one's health is essential. The study also revealed that those who practiced this were more knowledgeable about their health than those who did not. Therefore, the importance of having knowledge about your health will help you stay informed, ensuring an improvement in the quality of your health.

Also, it is important to mention that sharing your goals with an accountability partner can help you stay on track and improve your chances of achieving your goals.

There are numerous fitness journals in bookstores and on the internet. These journals are designed for short-term or long-term goals depending on your preference. You can find journals that will help keep track of your meals, calorie intake, measurements, liquid consumption, etc. Examples of fitness journals are Ban.do, Workout logbook & fitness journal, and Wellness planner.

CONCLUSION

Getting started on your fitness journey is simple as long as you have learned and incorporated all the aspects of losing weight. One important thing to get an understanding of is your body type. This will help you understand the interactions between the various facets of the body and how you can work with them to achieve your fitness goals.

Renowned American psychologist William Herbert Sheldon coined the word somatotypes to describe different structural body types — Ectomorph, Endomorph, and Mesomorph. This classification helps us understand that it is okay to react differently to a set of stimuli. Hence, you shouldn't expect to get the same result as someone else, even if you followed the same process.

So far, this book has covered three distinct ways of reducing weight - healthy eating, exercising, and Intermittent Fasting. We have explained how each aspect operates and integrates into the other for an efficient outcome. However, all of these still come down to knowing your particular body type. This will help you decide the most suitable method to apply to attain your ideal physique.

Key Points

➤ It is essential to identify and understand your body type, as it forms the foundation for your overall health.

➤ Your eating plan must be in line with your fitness goals.

➤ Have a meal plan to help you avoid unnecessary calories and unhealthy meals.

➤ Staying active is essential in your weight loss journey. However, you must ensure that you do it correctly and avoid over-exercising.

➤ Intermittent Fasting has its pros and cons; therefore, seek medical advice before exploring this option.

➤ Research your proposed weight-loss method before you begin to avoid common mistakes that will hinder your success

➤ Establishing goals for attaining your ideal physique is essential. However, it is what is key is that your goals are SMART!

➤ Keeping a fitness journal will help you stay on top of your fitness and health goals.

REFERENCES

Arenas, C. B. (2019, September 14). *Basal medabolic rate calculator*. Calculators.org. Retrieved from https://www.calculators.org/health/bmr.php.

Baier, L. (2020, April 18). *9 intermittent fasting mistakes (and how to avoid them!)*. A Sweet Pea Chef. Retrieved from https://www.asweetpeachef.com/intermittent-fasting-mistakes/.

Blair, S. N. (n.d.). *Overall conditioning*. Encyclopædia Britannica. Retrieved from https://www.britannica.com/topic/exercise-physical-fitness/Overall-conditioning.

Bridges, M. (2020, May 26). *Diet myths and facts: Medlineplus medical encyclopedia*. MedlinePlus. Retrieved from https://medlineplus.gov/ency/patientinstructions/000895.htm.

Dube, P. (2021, September 20). *Top 10 weight loss mistakes we all make*. HealthifyMe Blog. Retrieved from http://www.healthifyme.com/blog/top-10-weight-loss-mistakes-we-all-make/amp/.

Exercise. Encyclopedia of Children's Health. (n.d.).
    Retrieved from
    http://www.healthofchildren.com/E-
    F/Exercise.html.

Fletcher, J. (2020, March 9). *What to know about basal
    metabolic rate.* Medical News Today. Retrieved
    from medicalnewstoday.com/articles/basal-
    metabolic-rate.

Gunnars, K. (2020, April 21). *Intermittent fasting 101 – the
    ultimate beginner's guide.* Healthline. Retrieved
    from
    https://www.healthline.com/nutrition/intermittent-
    fasting-guide.

Gunnars, K. (2020, September 25). *How intermittent
    fasting can help you lose weight.* Healthline.
    Retrieved from
    https://www.healthline.com/nutrition/intermittent-
    fasting-and-weight-loss.

Gunnars, K. (2021, March 24). *6 popular ways to do
    intermittent fasting.* Healthline. Retrieved from
    https://www.healthline.com/nutrition/6-ways-to-
    do-intermittent-fasting.

Hill, C. (2014). *Gold's Gym blog | Fitness, nutrition ... -
    linglestown.* Retrieved from
    https://www.goldsgym.com/linglestown/blog/.

Intermittent fasting rules. OC Sports & Wellness. (2019, September 12). Retrieved from https://ocsportsandwellness.com/blog/intermitten t-fasting-rules/.

Legg, J. (2018). *Intermittent fasting: The complete beginner's guide to intermittent fasting for weight loss.*

Leonard, J. (2020, January 17). *16:8 intermittent fasting: Benefits, how-to, and tips.* Medical News Today. Retrieved from https://www.medicalnewstoday.com/articles/327 398.

Link, R. (2021, January 19). *What are the different stages of intermittent fasting?* Healthline. Retrieved from https://www.healthline.com/nutrition/stages-of-fasting.

Migala, J. (2019, November 20). *Endomorph Diet 101: Food List, Sample Menu, Benefits, More.* Everyday Health. Retrieved from https://www.everydayhealth.com/diet-nutrition/endomorph-diet/.

Migala, J., Rapaport, L., Kennedy, K., Manning, J., Migala, J., & Lawler, M. (2019, October 8). *Body type diet: Are you an ectomorph, mesomorph, or endomorph?* EverydayHealth.com. Retrieved from https://www.everydayhealth.com/diet-nutrition/body-type-diet-are-you-ectomorph-mesomorph-endomorph/.

Parkinson, N. (2018, February 27). *7 common workout mistakes to avoid.* Henry Ford LiveWell. Retrieved from http://www.henryford.com/blog/2018/02/7-common-workout-mistakes-avoid.

Petre, A., & Link, R. (2021, May 20). *Does calorie counting work? A critical look.* Healthline. Retrieved from https://www.healthline.com/nutrition/does-calorie-counting-work.

Pfaff, D. W. (n.d.). *Hormones, genes, and behaviour.*

Schlinger, A., (2021, September 24). *Trust me, a fitness journal will actually help you stick to your goals.* Women's Health. Retrieved from https://www.womenshealthmag.com/fitness/g25694091/fitness-journal/.

Somatotype and constitutional psychology - wikimili, the free encyclopedia. WikiMili.com. (n.d.). Retrieved from https://wikimili.com/en/Somatotype_and_constitutional_psychology.

Spritzler, F. (2021, August 10). *15 common mistakes when trying to lose weight.* Healthline. Retrieved from https://www.healthline.com/nutrition/weight-loss-mistakes.

Sylvie. (n.d.). *Intermittent Fasting According to Your Body Type: Fact or Fiction?* Fasting With Intention. Retrieved from fastingwithintention.com/intermittent-fasting-according-to-your-body-type/.

West, H. (2016, June 7). *Counting calories 101: How to count calories to lose weight.* Healthline. Retrieved from https://www.healthline.com/nutrition/counting-calories-101.

Williams, B. (2021, July 29). *Exercise for weight loss in 7 Days: Revving your fat burn to the Max.* BetterMe Blog. Retrieved from https://betterme.world/articles/exercise-for-weight-loss-in-7-days/.